God Bless you
for being a
part of Simon's
story. Love,
Sheryl Crosier

I Am Not a Syndrome - My Name is Simon

By "Trisomy Mom" Sheryl Crosier

Edited by Andy Knef

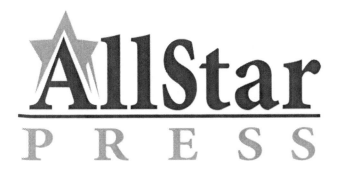

Published by

All Star Press

P.O. Box 2226

Tarpon Springs, FL 34689

www.allstarpress.com

ISBN: 978-1-937376-16-1

Library of Congress Control Number: 2012919653

Cover and jacket designed by All Star Press

Printed in the United States of America

A portion of proceeds from every sale of this book will go to **SOFT**, Support Organization for Trisomy 18, 13 and Related Disorders.

Go to Simonismyname.com for more information on Simon's story.

DEDICATION

To our beloved son, Simon Dominic Crosier, our precious loving little man, who encouraged so many to respect life. Thank you for being our shining light. Simon, you taught us compassion, patience, the understanding to live in the moment, and unconditional love. Our measurement of a life's value is in love.

I will always be thankful for the short time we had together and my life will never be the same. Because of you, Simon, I am no longer afraid to die.

As Jesus is the Author of salvation, through Him I will see you again.

"Always be prepared to make a defense to anyone who calls you to account for the hope that is in you, yet do it with gentleness and reverence." 1 Peter 3:15

Excerpts of What Others Have Said

"Be prepared for smiles, laughter and tears. This is a book well written by an amazing trisomy Mom!"

Alex Hauber
Executive director *Trisomy Advocacy Group*

"Sheryl Crosier's memoir, *I'm Not A Syndrome - My Name is Simon,* of her journey during her pregnancy and her infant son Simon's short but important life, is **a story of the heart and spirit.** It is also a story of the head that explores the capabilities and constraints of modern medicine and policy, parental rights and ethical decision making."

Pamela Healey, Ph.D. mother to Conor, Trisomy 18.

"This book is a love story shared by a family who believes that every life has purpose and worth."

Ann Barnes, RN and mother of Megan (1985-2004) born with Trisomy 18. Co-author of *Care of the Infant and Child with Trisomy 18 or 13* (2011)

"This is the heroic and gripping story of Sheryl and Scott Crosier as they struggle through the 88½ days of life given their son, Simon, born with Trisomy 18, a rare chromosomal abnormality.

Struggling with the fragility of Simon's life was one thing. However, struggling with the popular pragmatic culture that measures human life in terms of dollars rather than dignity, is quite another. Yet, all along the way, again and again, Sheryl and Scott discovered and were made disciples of Life. **This story celebrates both the pain and the joy of love!"**

Most Reverend Robert J. Hermann, Bishop Emeritus in Residence, *St. Louis Archdiocese of St. Louis*

"In reading '*I'm not a syndrome – My Name is Simon*,' you will get angry. You will get frustrated. You may shed a few tears. You may not believe that our lauded U.S. medical system could have the audacity to label a newborn baby as '*incompatible with life*.' And yet...

You will also smile with joy and laugh in surprise as you discover and wonder at the mystery of this unique child of God. **Simon spoke louder than some who have lived on this earth for decades!"**

Rev. Marty Guise
Executive Director
Lay Renewal Ministries

"There is so much more to this story than reading of a little boy's journey. It is learning about the legacy for which he was here. Simon will live on in the hearts of many and I feel he truly has a place in mine. I don't see Simon's life as a tragedy but as a beautiful blessing. God knew what he was doing when he helped to choose Simon's parents, for they are the ones who will bring his mission to its full potential."

Pat Jonas
President and Co-founder
Australian Rare Chromo Awareness Network (ARCAN)

"Your book is so wonderful Simon! You will help so many people, especially those who are gifted with children like you."

Tammy R Cowan
Imaging Miracles, Springfield Mo

"This book provides important insight and will allow providers to better understand parents who have children with Trisomy 13 and 18."

Barbara Farlow, BEngSci MBA, co-author of *The Experience of Parents of Children with Trisomy 13 and 18 in Social Networks*

"I'm Not a Syndrome — My Name Is Simon is an amazing combination of raw honesty, courage, determination, devotion and a whole lot of love."

Tanya Leckie
Gold Coast, Australia
(Mum to Cooper Trisomy 13 Mosaic)

"Sheryl's courage to confront a sometimes impassive medical system and to advocate on Simon's behalf is inspiring, and other families may find themselves borrowing her courage to do the same."

Sue Hall, MD, neonatologist and author of *For the Love of Babies*

"A beautiful testimony to the spirit of Simon and the lives that continue to be touched and transformed by his short life. Simon's gentleness, strength and presence remind us of the divine connection that knows no limits. What an extraordinary teacher!"

Pam Weiss MA
License Professional Counselor
Annie's Hope

CONTENTS

PREFACE

As eloquently spoken by many great writers and sages of the last century from the Dalai Lama to novelist Harper Lee, we can only know the life experiences of another human by "walking in their shoes." In times of crisis and life challenges, perhaps the only way to truly walk with another person is to take off our own "shoes" and humbly walk with our fellow traveler, arm in arm. Upon reading Sheryl Crosier's touching book, "I'm Not a Syndrome - My Name is Simon", that is your only choice — walk humbly with our fellow human. Ms. Crosier's story of her son, Simon, a boy with the Trisomy 18 syndrome who lived and died under the watchful and caring eyes of his parents and family, transforms the reader to the day-to-day events in Simon's short but meaningful life. By mindfully experiencing her words, the reader becomes in a matter of just a few pages — a fellow traveler.

As a pediatrician and specialist in medical genetics, I see the plight of families whose children have complex medical conditions daily, but — as pointed out poignantly by Crosier — at "the end of the day" we professionals go home, carry out the daily tasks of our everyday life, and move on. We recall the day's events on occasion, can be moved by them, and then proceed to the task at hand. But, not the parents of our "patients" — for these travelers it is 24/7 x 52. While in the past I have personally and professionally pondered this challenge of parents in this spot, reading "I'm Not a Syndrome - My Name is Simon" reminded me of this word-by-word, page-by-page in a deep and profound manner. By telling Simon's story, Ms. Crosier has captured this experience in a way that no medical account or case report of a genetic syndrome could even begin to touch. I feel it is important for those of us who have the privilege of caring for children with complex conditions to stop — listen — contemplate — take off our shoes — and walk with our fellow traveler. Sheryl Crosier's story of Simon allows us to do just that.

John C. Carey, MD, MPH

Department Of Pediatrics

University of Utah

ACKNOWLEDGEMENTS

I wish to express my heartfelt gratitude to my son, Simon. For you showed me your signs and guided me as I wrote your book. You also put in my path the people you wanted to be a part of your book.

Thank you to our dear friend and special education teacher Krista for encouraging me to write this book. Thank you for your help in reviewing my early work as I was so emotionally raw.

I also want to thank Cynthia Wellington, dear friend and Christian author, who reviewed chapters and assisted in implementing Biblical truths.

Particularly, I am forever grateful for my editor, Andy Knef, who has traveled this journey with me. Our Lord placed Andy in our family for a reason and we are so blessed to have such a wonderful friend.

Thank you to Dr. Debbie Bruns, Investigator of TRIS and author. We are honored to have Simon included in your TRIS project and your book, "Feeding Challenges in Young Children." If it were not for you, I would not have attended my first SOFT conference in Chicago.

Thank you to our reading panel, Ann Barnes, Pam Healey, Barb Farlow, Marty Guise, Jeanne Maher, Louise Lord, Maggie Weik and Faye Kaufman.

Thank you to our proofreaders, Sheila Stock and Margaret Wilke.

Thank you to Dr. Steve Cantrell and Peggy. We know our sons are buddies in heaven. We are always on the lookout for "Simon signs" and "Ryan reminders." It seems like we have been friends for a long time, or should I say "family."

Thank you to the entire SOFT family. Without this organization, we would feel so alone. You are all so special to our entire family. I look forward to many more SOFT reunions.

Thank you to Simon's special nurses and doctors — for he knows those of you who were his advocates. We pray that other trisomy children in your care may be blessed and looked at as an individual and not a syndrome.

For all of you who made Simon's first memorial golf tournament such a huge success. Spring Creek Golf Course will always be sacred ground. Thank you Seneca, Kansas.

Thank you to Dr. Hall, Neonatologist, author and friend who spent many hours with me and allowed me to introduce Simon to her. Thank you for supporting Simon's golf tournament and for being an advocate for Trisomy children.

Thank you to Dr. Carey, Pediatrician and Geneticist, for your kindness in reviewing Simon's medical records and sharing your wisdom of trisomy and genetics with us. We are all so blessed to have you in the Trisomy community for over 25 years.

Thank you to Dr. Braddock, Pediatrician and Geneticist for reviewing Scott's karyotype and offering feedback on this book. St. Louis is blessed to have you here.

Thank you to Troy and Judy Popielarz for allowing me to walk with you on your journey — from the prenatal diagnosis of Trisomy 18, throughout your pregnancy and the arrival of your son, Nathaniel Troy Popielarz. Nathaniel will always be in my heart. I will forever cherish the priceless time with my God Child.

Thank you to our family and friends. We will always remember the love and support you gave us and I believe Simon will too. Thank you for walking beside us in our grief journey and understanding that grief will be ours for a lifetime until we are reunited with Simon and all of our children. Thanks for supporting the mission to keep Simon's legacy alive.

Most of all I want to thank and express my love for my awesome husband, Scott and my three precious sons, Samuel, Sean and Simon and our six beautiful daughters, Sophia, Hope, Sarah, Joy Therese, Mae and Faith living in heaven. My family gave me both the motivation and drive to continue on with this book. I love you all.

INTRODUCTION

This book is written for those who'll forever love and honor Simon and for those who are advocates for special needs children and the unborn. In these pages, you'll learn about the battle Simon's family fought to defend their son's life and dignity.

"Battle" and "fought" are strong words. I don't use them lightly. Our efforts to do our very best for our physically threatened son were the most difficult experience we've ever encountered. At times, in the heat of our struggle to get our perspective across to well-meaning medical professionals who literally kept Simon alive with their expertise, we disagreed on care approaches and bedside manner. Those differences in outlook were sometimes profound; but never, I believe, based on lack of skill or best intentions to do what these caregivers felt were in our son's medical interest.

We found many among Simon's medical team to be kind, generous and straightforward in the most helpful ways imaginable. Sadly, a few seemed eager to help us get past what they viewed as a tragic, but unchangeable, fate that random chance and a chromosomal abnormality had wrought. I'm sure they wanted to make the right decision. I'm convinced they tried to do their best, and if I misunderstood any of their words or actions in re-telling Simon's story, my mistakes are born of a mother's grief and stress during the hardest of times.

But there is something that should be very clear as you read this account. My family doesn't believe in random chance. Simon had a name. He also had a divine purpose! My family, as well as countless others we've met in the trisomy community, believe the best interests of society are always bound up in caring for and valuing the most vulnerable of its citizens.

This story is Simon's story, and his family's story. Others faced with these daunting circumstances will travel a different path. We believe that Simon still has lessons to share for those who value the dignity of every life and the potential of every child to change the world with God-given talents and an unbowed eternal soul.

Please walk our personal journey with us as we persevere through the agony of six miscarriages, only to grasp the joy of carrying Simon to his birth by cesarean section on Sept. 7, 2010. We'll take you through Simon's Trisomy 18 diagnosis and give you a glimpse of his strength and unique spirit. He captured our family's unconditional love with his big, lovely eyes and knowing expression.

Finally, we'll paint a brief picture of our everyday lives in the present as we continue to grow and learn from our time with our precious son. It's a reality without our Simon physically here on Earth — but surrounded by his discernible presence in heaven.

Disclaimer:

Some names of people and facilities have been changed in this account. Those instances are marked in the text by a *. All other names and facility references are accurate. All changes are at the request of the person referenced or to preclude categorical inferences that the author does not mean to imply.

CHAPTER ONE

He knit you in my womb

"Dear Lord, I pray that I will not get pregnant if I am not able to bring a baby to term and hold our child in my arms." — Prayer said nightly in preparation for Simon's birth

Losing a child is a pain so deep that is difficult for anyone to grasp. It can be like falling down a chasm that seems to have no bottom. The chasm is lined with thorn branches that scrape and pull at your skin when you remember what you have lost.

My husband, Scott, and I lost six children through miscarriage. With each loss, the sting of pain was greater. The counsel from well-meaning family members and friends became more difficult to hear. After we lost our daughter, Faith, to miscarriage in September of 2008, we rid our home of most of our baby items.

But still…

Each day, I would read and pray Psalm 139:13-16. *For you created my inmost being. You knit me together in my mother's womb…All the days ordained for me were written in your book before one of them came to be.* Even in the valley, I looked to God for His help and direction.

Then, in early 2010, we learned we were expecting. Our baby's due date was September 22, 2010. Scott and I, along with our two living sons —Samuel, age 7, and Sean, age 5 — were filled with joy and yet terrified at the thought of losing another baby.

On September 7, 2010, at 5:40 p.m., we heard the first cry of Simon Dominic Crosier as he entered this world. On December 3, 2010, the tears poured forth from our eyes and others as Simon left this world for his eternal home.

Although his life was short, Simon brought so much love and joy and touched so many hearts that his story demanded to be told. As you journey with us through the pages of this book, we hope you will gain an understanding of a life-challenging syndrome called Trisomy 18. In the eyes of some in the medical community, a child with this syndrome is considered "*incompatible with life*."

But God did not bless us with a syndrome. God blessed us with a son. His name was Simon.

Through the pages of this book, we want to tell you Simon's story. It is a story filled with joy and sorrow. It is a story filled with compassion and outrage. It is a story of a child knit together by the Hand of God. Each of his days was written and ordained.

Thank you for being a part of Simon's story.

CHAPTER TWO

The battle begins

I picked up the book The Help *by Kathryn Stockett. At that time I had no way of knowing how much this tale of African Americans' lonely battle against prejudice and misguided conventional wisdom would have corollaries to my own family's struggles.*

After the loss of our fourth baby, my doctor advised a karyotype analysis for Scott and me. Karyotype refers to a person's full set of chromosomes. Each person has two strands that are woven together and determine a number of factors, including gender. In this karyotype analysis, doctors conducted a genetic comparison of a "normal" karyotype with our samples for any abnormalities.

The following analysis of Scott's karyotype is taken almost directly from notes that were shared with me after a genetic counseling session I attended on March 11, 2009. In addition, Dr. Steven Braddock, MD, the St. Louis area's leading authority on trisomy-related genetic abnormalities, reviewed Scott's records. Dr. Braddock is the director of Medical Genetics at Cardinal Glennon Children's Medical Center in St. Louis

According to Dr. Braddock's careful explanation in the summer of 2012, my husband's X-chromosome strand is structured so a portion of the chromosome is inverted, or "flipped." Called a pericentric inversion, this structure goes from the p21.2 region through the q13 region (p stands for the short arm of a chromosome and q for the long arm). Since the total amount of genetic material Scott possesses is normal, he never presented any secondary physical or developmental problems.

Despite Scott's good health, carriers of chromosome inversions may be at increased risk to have chromosomally abnormal children due to the production of egg or sperm cells that have an unbalanced amount of chromosome material present. In our case, the risk might be higher for a female child than a male because a boy wouldn't receive an X-chromosome from Scott. Dr. Braddock tells us the best risk estimate for an unbalanced chromosome makeup in an offspring is about 10-15 percent with each pregnancy. It's not known what portion of those pregnancies would result in a miscarriage versus a liveborn infant with abnormalities.

Our hearts were filled with joy as we discovered on May 6, 2010 that we were having a boy! During the ultrasound at nearby Missouri General Hospital* in St. Louis, we immediately felt this news lessened our odds of another miscarriage. We believed, finally, our worries would be over. We thought we might be able to relax, enjoy this pregnancy and joyfully prepare for the arrival of our little boy in September.

At our first ultrasound, we encountered our first conflict when our doctors suggested an amniocentesis. We refused. Despite their concern that something could potentially be wrong with our unborn son, we knew we would never terminate the pregnancy. Simon's due date was September 22, 2010. Our two living sons —Samuel, age 7, and Sean, age 5 — shared our anticipation.

The ultrasound doctor Dr. Rodgers* seemed to be a knowledgeable woman, but short on empathy. She noted our little boy's hands were clenched. A cleft lip and clenched hands are potential signs of a genetic abnormality. The sonographer and doctor tried to determine if our baby's tiny fingers were overlapped, another sign of chromosomal issues. Scott and I were very unhappy that these medical professionals were talking about our baby as if we weren't even in the room. We were scared!

Then something wonderful happened to relieve our panic. Scott later told me that on his way back to work he felt Jesus' peace. At that moment, the Holy Spirit revealed to my husband our baby boy's full name — Simon Dominic Crosier. It's a wonderful, strong name with a Biblical foundation and the original name of the apostle who is the cornerstone of Christ's church on Earth.

Throughout the ordeal of my miscarriages, counseling had been a blessing to me. I continued seeing a counselor during my pregnancy with Simon. At first it was for reassurance and anxiety reduction, even though things were going well. Soon, it was to help me navigate while information and suspicions were voiced and tests were suggested. Before this ultrasound, everything had seemed fine — except my anxiety about miscarrying again.

My obstetrician had described Simon's progress this way: "Everything looks fine, nice growth. I worry about some of my patients; you're not one of them." When she added that I might consider reading a good novel, I picked up the book *The Help* by Kathryn Stockett. At that time I had no way of knowing this tale of African Americans' lonely battle against prejudice and misguided conventional wisdom would have corollaries to my own family's struggles with advocating for Simon.

I also called the genetic counselor. After reviewing Simon's ultrasounds, she said our results didn't indicate Down syndrome or Trisomy 18. She added, "There is no evidence of birth defects at this time." Then she said something that unnerved me despite her calm demeanor. "We got a suboptimal view of the heart and need the front face picture of the lip and the chin. It's not unusual to go back for more pictures," she said, but I knew that almost nothing had ever gone the "usual" way in our efforts to build our family.

My counselor, Gail, insisted that each pregnancy is different. Since Gail's specialty was reproductive health, many of her patients were women who had lost babies to miscarriages, stillbirth or infant death. "That's history," she would say about our six miscarriages. "This pregnancy is separate. Don't try to connect them."

By this time our boys were making comments about how Mommy's tummy was getting bigger. We hadn't told the boys about Simon's arrival because we wanted to protect them from any potential hurt. Of all my miscarriages, they only knew about Sophia, our first lost baby. We decided to tell the boys about their siblings in heaven when they got older. To deflect questions, I told Samuel and Sean I was going to see my doctor in a couple of weeks to see why Mommy's tummy was so big.

After my doctor's appointment, we told the boys about our news. If Samuel knew all along, he sweetly played along for his brother's benefit. I added, "The doctor said that the baby is really healthy and expects him to be just fine." They were so excited. When Samuel said "I knew it; I told you there was a baby in your belly," we responded that he would surely be a doctor someday. Then Sean said, "Finally I get to be a big brother. Can we name the baby?" Scott and I immediately said, "No, we already have a name for him. It's Simon Dominic Crosier."

Our family is all S's — even our pet fish, Sonic Bolt and Shadow Rocket. You can see that our choice to keep Simon's naming an adult decision was probably wise.

The unbridled joy of our sons about the news was one thing, but we were also dealing with a lack of support from those we hoped we could count on. Loved ones expected us to rejoice at the pregnancies of others while tempering our own enthusiasm about Simon's arrival. The constant warnings to proceed with caution — "Don't get your hopes too high" —

became oppressive and discouraging. Worse, these inconsiderate words made us feel alone.

As we moved some family members and former close friends to our outer circle of trust, we had to accept that estrangement was probably the best solution. We simply ignored the naysayers and "boxed" the resentment. I give credit to my counselor for offering me the visual: "box it up." That image got my attention immediately. Down the road I knew I would have to deal with these feelings but now my family needed to move forward. The reality of our situation wouldn't allow for toxic people who had never shown compassion when we lost six babies to miscarriages — toxic people like my own relatives.

CHAPTER THREE

Hoping for the best

"Thank you, God," I said again, nearly jumping with joy. Our prayer of closing that space in Simon's heart, which had left a hole in all of our hearts, was answered.

Trying to relax took tremendous effort. I had made it through the miscarriage stage, but now I worried about what might happen during the second trimester. I have friends who have lost babies at this point. I found it almost impossible not to think about them. I met many of these friends in my grief support group. This is a group of wounded faith seekers I hold close to my heart and pray for regularly. They helped me understand my own history was the basis for my fear.

My counselor and I talked often about honest self-evaluation: I was a healthy pregnant woman, keeping myself in a balanced state of spiritual, physical and mental wellbeing. I tried not to give in to fear. I tried hard, but my peace of mind only lasted so long. My pregnancy was a reminder of multiple traumas. Perhaps, I thought, my anxiety reflected the physical reminder of my stretched stomach — enlarged so many times with tragic results. Whatever my future, I had to be involved in managing it. Whatever my fate, I was in charge — with Jesus by my side.

As we left for our family vacation in Gulf Shores, Alabama, the soothing ocean vistas of our annual getaway destination began to fade — replaced by my worries over the pending follow-up ultrasound on June 7. We prayed as a family every night, laying our collective hands on Simon in my belly — asking the Lord for a healthy baby boy.

I couldn't wait for the ultrasound. Wouldn't it be great to have this trial past? I looked forward to the comfort of good news with my follow-up in the rear-view mirror.

The day of the second ultrasound finally arrived. My obstetrician, Dr. Seti*, had requested another ultrasound doctor since we found our first physician lacking in bedside manner and professionalism. To our surprise, the requested doctor wasn't available, and we endured Dr. Rodgers again. On the positive side, the sonogram immediately revealed that previously identified cysts of the choroid plexus (fluid-containing spaces within the brain) were gone. "Thank you, God!" Unfortunately, Dr. Rodgers' outlook wasn't equally improved. We told her how excited we were that the brain cysts were gone. We praised God for that. Her response: "Not a big deal that they're gone now since I saw the cysts initially within a certain window. That's what matters."

As I lay on the table undergoing the procedure, Dr. Rodgers and the sonographer conducted their own detached discussion of Simon's possible bilateral cleft lip and the potential hole in his heart. She referred us to St. Louis Children's Hospital to have a fetal echocardiogram conducted by a highly respected pediatric cardiologist.

The next day we arrived for our appointment at Children's Hospital. Two sonographers with 42 years of combined experience and the cardiologist, Dr. Johnson, found no defects with Simon's heart. The doctor explained additional tissue could have closed up the apparent hole. "Thank you, God," I said again, nearly jumping with joy. Our prayer to close that space in Simon's heart, which had left a hole in all of our hearts, was answered. We enjoyed some peace of mind about our baby for the first time in weeks. As I left Dr. Johnson's office, one of the sonographers, said, "You have a beautiful baby." I so wanted to cry! This was the first time a professional who had viewed one of Simon's sonograms complimented our baby. Maybe Simon did have a bilateral cleft lip, but the wonders of modern plastic surgery are incredible — even for tiny infants. It didn't matter anyway. We would love him just the same, cleft lip or not. A detail still lingered ominously in our minds. We wondered if his clenched fists could still mean he had Trisomy 18.

Maybe Simon's hands were clenched, but didn't the doctor tell us that clenched fists are fairly new criteria for identifying birth defects? Dr. Seti agreed with us that Dr. Rodgers showed insensitivity. She also disagreed with her evaluation of the brain cysts window, assuring us that this development was indeed "good news." I was grateful, but I couldn't help asking myself: Are they going to pick up anything else with future tests based on my history? How can I keep my anxiety level down? I have already undergone multiple ultrasounds. Because of all of my miscarriages, I'm under a microscope, and so is my precious Simon.

More difficult news came later that month. A relative sent a card informing our family that even though she had severed her relationship with us the previous Christmas, she wanted another chance. Despite the fact that she had never been supportive through our miscarriages, I decided to cautiously allow her back into our lives. Scott had misgivings, but I believed she missed us, and I wanted to go forward. I did set the ground rules: Our children are sensitive, and impulsive words can hurt badly, I reminded her sternly. Don't say outrageous things to get our attention. Respect the rules we've set up for our own peace of mind. We won't be yelled at or cursed at anymore. We have boundaries.

As we moved forward with the pregnancy, my stomach seemed to grow daily. My overriding goal was to hold my anxiety in check. At this point, I was on modified bed rest because of my blood pressure. Instructed to stay inactive, I had plenty of time to evaluate the situation. My growing baby had active kick counts. His organs looked good. His heart rate was perfect. Top specialists in the field of neonatal care monitored Simon's progress. The observations about his clenched fists and cleft lip were speculative. It was certainly in the realm of possibility that he was perfectly okay. Still, my mind backtracked. I struggled to tell myself that doubts were outside our control. I tried to remember that unless you have evidence to the contrary, the truth is established by medical facts.

We wanted Simon to sense our excitement and love for him — not our worries. Samuel and Sean read him books and sang to their brother. Every night we continued to pray over our little boy and praise and thank God for removing the cysts from his brain and closing the hole in his heart. We continued to look to the day when Simon would leave the warmth of Mommy's womb and take his place in all our arms. Scott's Mom, Grandma Lois, had a quilt made for Simon. This was her personal act of faith, hope and love.

Scott was sure he had seen Simon's hands open during my May sonogram, but Dr. Rodgers quickly dismissed Scott's observation. She'd have to see it herself, she said. When Dr. Seti advised getting a second opinion, we were grateful. Caregivers at Missouri General had eagerly recommended doing an amniocentesis with the conditional recommendation that we consider terminating the pregnancy. These so-called compassionate professionals related that some parents request an abortion because their baby has a cleft lip. Our reply was instantaneous: "No, we will keep our baby, no matter what! We will never terminate!" Scott and I are proudly pro-life. Each human being is born with intrinsic value, and deserves to be treated with dignity. At this point, our caregivers directed us to St. Paul's Hospital*. We knew that if God allowed Simon to have Trisomy 18, St. Paul's had a level-three neonatal unit and was well equipped to handle babies with these special needs.

Doctors discovered my blood pressure was elevated. We wondered if this could be an early start of preeclampsia. I endured this condition at the end of my pregnancies with Samuel and Sean. I was induced early with both, so I was very relieved when a urine sample revealed no protein and therefore made the diagnosis of preeclampsia less likely. The doctor's advice was concise, but not easy to execute: Rest often; stay off my feet and elevate them; no activity; and avoid the heat. I was told to monitor my blood pressure two times a day. Count kicks only two times a day to avoid needless anxiety. Doctors included some good news. Simon's fingers didn't appear to be overlapped.

I went to Gail for counseling weekly, always battling my fears. I needed to keep talking about my worries, and Gail continued to walk by my side on my journey. She understood the medical terminology, and had even seen babies with Trisomy 18, including a handsome, precious little boy named Ryan, who I would come to know later.

The next comprehensive ultrasound took place at St. Paul's one week later. Simon's heart was examined closely. I mentioned that we had a fetal echocardiogram at Children's and doctors believed they were seeing tissue, not a hole, in little Simon's heart. When I met Dr. Heddiger* for the first time, he greeted me with the three most terrible words I had ever heard. He said, "There are problems." He explained Simon's hands were clenched and they hadn't seen them open, despite what Scott had noted. There was still no overlapping of the fingers. This was a good sign because Trisomy 18 is typically characterized by this physical characteristic. Dr. Heddiger did observe the bilateral cleft lip, but the palate looked intact. As I lay there in near panic mode, doctors started looking at Simon's heart again. I was shaken and anxious. They said they needed Dr. Johnson's report from Children's Hospital. I wondered why I had to explain the report, which said Simon's heart was okay. I found myself screaming, "Please stop this ultrasound!"

Dr. Heddiger then scheduled a three-dimensional ultrasound of Simon's face and cleft lip. Again, the sonographer was far from compassionate. As she was looking at Simon's face, I asked if everything was okay. She responded curtly, "No it's not okay — don't you know he has a bilateral cleft lip?" I desperately told myself that he would be fine. We would love Simon cleft lip and all. How could anyone terminate a baby because he had a cleft lip? I guess our society demands our babies be "picture perfect" when they're delivered. We're not part of that society. We didn't care about his cleft lip. We just wanted our Simon.

My anxiety continued to rise. The sonographer left the room. A resident was now practicing on me as we waited for my doctor to come in. The resident asked if I was okay and my pent-up frustration exploded, "No, my blood pressure must be through the roof and my anxiety level is high!" I lay helplessly on that table as she kept rolling the wand over my round pregnant belly looking at Simon. When I finally told her to "Get out and go practice on someone else," she left quickly.

Dr. Gilbride*, a partner in Dr. Heddiger's practice, arrived announcing that Scott and I had decided not to have an amniocentesis. "We'll treat this baby as if there is no chromosomal abnormality," she said. "But we'll also be prepared for the worst case." I must admit I found something troubling in the phrase "treat this baby." Did she mean, "treat" clinically or something else? Dr. Gilbride reassured me that my baby's chromosome-related risk factors had nothing to do with my age. "We did see some extra amniotic fluid, but nothing to worry about," she added.

On July 15, Simon weighed 2 pounds, 9 ounces. The doctor showed us a chart placing these numbers firmly in the normal range. We had hope!

Samuel and Sean were always smiling and giggling when they felt Simon kicking. Every night we read Samuel and Sean their devotional and prayed over Simon. Sean said his own prayer. He knew that God put tissue on Simon's heart so he prayed, "Dear Jesus please put tissue paper on Simon's lip. Amen." We couldn't help laughing. We told Sean about the medical meaning of "tissue" in the body.

Dr. Heddiger would deliver our precious boy. We stayed with him because Dr. Seti referred him and because he had earned a reputation as an excellent high-risk doctor. The fact that Dr. Heddiger was on staff at St. Paul's — with its level-3 NICU — also made a positive difference in our minds. My personal relationship with Dr. Heddiger, after many appointments, was much less positive. After all the ultrasounds and tests and prior miscarriage traumas, why was I being robbed of the joy of this pregnancy? Not just me, but also my husband and two little boys. Why couldn't this be a blissful time in our lives? My doctor was not naturally upbeat or optimistic. His typical response was, "What do you want to hear, Sheryl?"

I reminded myself that Dr. Heddiger was a very good doctor and surgeon. I tried to put his personality aside. My anxiety was growing. I felt deeply shaken. I knew that my hypertension was dangerous for Simon and me. Maybe my own anxiety was making Dr. Heddiger uncomfortable, I worried.

Dr. Heddiger recommended we set up an interdisciplinary medical team to be ready just in case. If we truly needed a cardiologist, we would need a St. Paul's specialist.

A pediatric cardiologist at St. Paul's, Dr. Zandra*, performed another fetal echocardiogram. He found a very small hole in Simon's heart. It's called a Ventricular Septal Defect or VSD. This unwelcome news upset me further. Were we dealing with another marker for Trisomy 18? Dr. Zandra disagreed. "No, not a marker, this is so minor," he said. "This is nothing to worry about."

VSDs are found in only two percent of all babies, but the condition is not always a Trisomy 18 indicator. Dr. Zandra insisted that despite Simon's bilateral cleft lip and clenched fists, the VSD finding was "minor." He even indicated that it might close before Simon was born and, in any case, could be corrected after his birth by surgery. I took this positive approach to heart. Simon's heart and cleft lip need not mean the worst. There was also no undue stress on the heart for either a vaginal or C-section delivery, Doctor Zandra added. He was confident in his opinion: "No Trisomy 18." When I asked him if I would bring this baby to term, he assured us, "Yes, his heart is good!"

The next day Dr. Zandra called me and said, "Great news! After you left my office yesterday, I looked even closer and I saw tissue growing. There is a very good chance the hole will close by the time he is born."

The next evening, I was driving to my counselor's office listening to the Christian radio station. The announcers were talking about decisive faith. Choose faith no matter what, they said. Just then I turned the corner and saw the most beautiful rainbow. I believe this was God's promise to me. I had to continue keeping the faith. At that moment, I felt God's presence. My heart was filled with hope.

I decided to choose medical professionals who were positive, supportive and compassionate. Dr. Heddiger was one part of Simon's care team. But he was not the master of this ceremony. Simon Dominic Crosier was the only emcee I cared about. We awaited his debut with open arms. "Don't focus on Dr. Heddiger," I told myself. "Shrink him down because you've blown him up and he's taking up too much of the picture." You can get certain things from a skilled surgeon. But if he just doesn't have the other stuff, like compassion, I needed to draw those qualities from other professionals. I knew, however, I would insist on holding specialists to the standard of searching scrupulously for answers to questions about Simon's status.

Dr. Heddiger had no filter. I'll never forget the day he casually mentioned Scott's inversion as a crossover of two chromosomes. I looked at him so confused. A crossover? He said to me, "You know, you've heard this before." I then called the same genetic counselor at Missouri General who had explained the meaning of Scott's inversion of the X chromosome. She said, "This is highly unlikely to involve a crossover." This kind of structural abnormality between an X and Y chromosome is very unlikely and an exchange of genetic material is equally rare, she added. She questioned why Dr. Heddiger would even bring it up.

Simon would enter this world shortly. We wanted to be excited and positive and welcome him. The doctors were always vague about his condition. I chose to process this information in a confident way. Dr. Heddiger said I was stable. I was also pretty far along. This was the time to take control of my fear. Things continued to go well through July. Simon's heartbeat continued in the 138-beats-per-minute range, which is considered strong. Unfortunately, I had sleep issues. I'd wake up around 3 a.m., and didn't fall back asleep until 5 or 6 a.m. Then, I was up with the boys around 7 -7:30 a.m. I talked to Dr. Heddiger's nurse about a sedative. I tried melatonin one night, and it didn't help, so I decided I'd just do without much sleep on some nights. Dr. Heddiger assured me that my sleep problems had nothing physically to do with Simon's possible cleft lip. I was put on baby aspirin to protect my heart before I got pregnant. I remained on it until about the 35th week of pregnancy.

In late July we met with Dr. Rivers*, the plastic surgeon. He said he reviewed the 3D ultrasound and confirmed that Simon had a mild bilateral cleft lip and an intact palate. He called this "great news" because cleft palate is usually associated with chromosomal abnormalities. He added that he could conduct plastic surgery on the cleft lip when Simon was eight to ten weeks old.

We also learned in our online research that cleft lips are more common in boys. They occur in one of 600-700 babies and are the third most common birth defect. In Simon's case, with just his lip affected, and no split in the gum, one surgery at age eight to ten weeks could repair the damage. By the time he was six to seven years old, we would have to tell him that he was born with a cleft lip. We wouldn't know until he was born if there was a soft cleft palate. While his hard palate seemed to be intact, ultrasounds don't show the soft palate or soft gum line. This was good news even if there were complications. It's nearly impossible to pinpoint why a child is born with a cleft lip. Since Simon was my ninth pregnancy, maybe it was just the random chance that his lip was cleft. Dr. Rivers said we might need the NICU for feeding issues. Still, we considered it great news that Simon merely had a cleft lip and not Trisomy 18.

In July we also met with Dr. Pang*, a neonatologist at St. Paul's NICU. Dr. Pang was very kind. He asked, "Do you have a name for him yet?" When I told him Simon's name, Dr. Pang said, "If Simon just has a cleft lip, he'll possibly be in the NICU for tube feeding. We'll assess Simon when he's born, but we won't know until then precisely what he needs."

Dr. Pang again assured us that fingers in babies with Trisomy 18 are usually overlapped. These babies also often have heart problems and apnea. After reviewing all of the notes and ultrasounds, he advised that we talk about Simon as if he was otherwise healthy and had only a cleft lip. Melanie Ward*, the patient support nurse, was also at the meeting. Dr. Pang kept referring to our baby using his beautiful name Simon, reminding us that Simon was a little person, not a condition. We set up an appointment for a tour of the NICU.

A few weeks later, when we toured the old NICU, all the babies were in the same area. There were no private rooms.

We noticed the sizes of the babies. We tried to figure out how much Simon would weigh. Melanie explained that the new NICU with private rooms and animal name pods would be complete before Simon's arrival. The pods had names like Giraffe, Elephant, Panda and Koala. It sounded nice, but we were still sure Simon wouldn't need the NICU. If he did, it would be for feeding issues and not for conditions related to Trisomy 18.

Melanie agreed that the information from Drs. Zandra and Rivers and the previous ultrasounds were very positive indicators. One experienced sonographer pointed out that Simon's fingers and hands were opening. Finally, someone could confirm what Scott saw. Melanie even said, "Tally it up. There are more positives than negatives." She said the NICU gets a couple of babies with cleft lips a year and sees one or two Trisomy 18 babies a year. About 10,000 babies a year are delivered at St. Paul's.

I underwent a non-stress test in early August. The test monitors fetal activity and movement in addition to fetal heart tones. Simon did awesome! *Jean, the sonographer thought he was still in breech position. I thought of Simon as a tiny gymnast who flipped every week. When the sonographer did the ultrasound she concluded that Simon had "flipped" out of the breech position and my amniotic fluid supply was generous. When she saw Simon's face, she said, "He's smiling at you. He has your chin, so cute, so sweet. And look at his button nose." She took his picture and typed "Baby Simon" on it.

Scott and I cried tears of joy. We were so touched that someone called our little Simon sweet and cute. All our descriptions until then seemed to be based on scrutinizing all his possible problems. Then Jean said, "Look at his fingers. His hand is like this, now. He's hitchhiking." Alleluia! Scott and I hugged Jean. We were so excited.

We decided Dr. Heddiger was outnumbered. By valuing the positive opinions of all the medical professionals on the team, we could best reduce our anxiety. As my counselor said, "Go with what you know." God had placed many positive compassionate people in our lives. We needed to keep faith and hope.

During the following week's ultrasound to check Simon's position and amniotic fluid we learned Simon was reaching for his toes. The sonographer told us that he was practicing breathing on his own, and that this was a good reflex. When we saw Dr. Heddiger in the hall, I told him I could measure my stomach at home. "I'm not having any more comprehensive ultrasounds after today," I said forcefully. Scott couldn't resist asking Dr. Heddiger, "If we had an ultrasound machine at home, would you believe us about Simon?" Dr. Heddiger could only answer, "Okay, we're close enough to delivery."

When we entered the room for the last comprehensive ultrasound the sonographer did many measurements. She said Simon was small, about 2 pounds, 11 ounces, but told us not to worry. The placenta looked good, and the oxygen distribution to his brain also seemed on track. Dr. Gillbride came in and agreed that Simon was small. He was below the 10th percentile, but she told us not to worry. She predicted a delivery at the end of August at about six pounds. After we left the room, we were at the desk making our next appointment when the sonographer walked by. She said, "What a beautiful baby." How wonderful! Even if, in her own mind, she feared something was wrong with Simon, she kindly offered us this beautiful, simple compliment. Then she added, "Don't worry; some of my own children were small."

How could we not worry about Simon's size? A family friend, Carla, did her own research and found that the normal range for babies at the end of 34 weeks is 3.5 to 5 pounds. She also found a study showing that garlic can increase fetal growth.

That's all I needed to hear; I swallowed garlic cloves. Since I had been struggling with anxiety, any positive news went a long way. My counselor, Gail, constantly reminded me not to borrow trouble, but I kept thinking about how close we were to delivery. I questioned my decision to forego another ultrasound.

The only thing we really knew at this point was that Simon had a cleft lip and might be small. I wanted to say to Dr. Heddiger, "I sometimes find it difficult to digest things you've thrown out there. As a prospective mom who's had many disappointments, can you help calm me? Instead, you make me more anxious." His medical assistant, however, was very kind and compassionate. "We've seen cleft lips before," she said. "Don't worry. You and the baby will be fine."

When my blood pressure reading rose to 170/110 at my next appointment, Dr. Heddiger asked to see me. He suggested we deliver Simon soon because of his "growth restriction." Later, I learned the medical community modified this term from "intrauterine growth retardation." We didn't find his remarks reassuring. With my obvious anxiety about delivery, why couldn't he just say "small?" Was something wrong? Dr. Heddiger added that whatever the baby's position during labor, we'd deliver that way. Too risky to turn Simon, and, of course, he didn't want to take any chances.

CHAPTER FOUR

Simon's here!

We had prayed every night for a healthy baby with the correct number of chromosomes. But now our baby had Trisomy 18, and we wondered, "Why God?"

We kept repeating all the positives — heart good, "No Trisomy 18," as Dr. Zandra said. We saw Simon's hands open several times and so did the sonographer. All of Simon's non-stress tests earned passing grades indicating Simon was reacting to his environment. Dr. Rivers would examine Simon after he was born and determine the plastic surgery plan.

The evening of my scheduled induction, our whole family went to dinner at Imo's pizza in Webster. As we were leaving, I noticed a baby boy, six months old, with a cleft lip. I introduced myself and told the family that my baby Simon would have a bilateral cleft lip and I was going to the hospital in a few hours to deliver him. The little boy's name was Parker. He was this couple's first child. He needed to wait for surgery for his cleft because of a heart condition. This meeting was no coincidence — it was a *Godincidence*. During my pregnancy, I heard of people who had their clefts repaired, but I yearned to see a baby with a cleft lip. God answered my prayer. Other children with cleft lips overcame that challenge. Maybe there was still a chance that God would put tissue paper on Simon's lip.

We arrived at the hospital at about 8:30 p.m. on September 6, 2010 (ironically, Labor Day). Dr. Heddiger wanted to deliver

Simon sooner than his due date of September 22. Valerie*, our dear friend and a nurse anesthetist at St. Paul's, helped ensure we were given a comfortable delivery room. Also, Valerie did all she could to provide me with a delivery nurse with compassion. We met Colleen*. Another *Godincidence*! Colleen's friend has four children and all four were born with cleft lips. Colleen and I talked about everything we had gone through during the pregnancy and how things were looking very positive. I told Colleen the doctors had noted signs of markers for Trisomy 18, but most had disappeared, except the cleft lip. Since Dr. Rivers identified the palate as primarily associated with chromosomal abnormalities, not the lip, we were optimistic. We repeated our plan that if Simon's mild bilateral cleft lip required assistance in the NICU it would be only for feeding issues. Colleen listened intently and told me not to worry about Dr. Heddiger — sometimes known around the hospital as "Dr. Doom and Gloom."

Colleen added that if Simon had Trisomy 18, medical professionals wouldn't typically monitor his heart rate. She continued saying these babies tend to show signs of distress during labor. Since Simon was on the monitor and he had passed all of his non-stress tests, things were looking good. But why, I had to ask myself, didn't they monitor the Trisomy 18 baby's heart rate? Was it because they figured the baby wouldn't live? This sounded like these babies were "treated" unfairly. I was disturbed by that suggestion.

Several hours after being induced, doctors noticed some deceleration of Simon's heart rate. We had made it clear that any signs of distress should lead to a C-section. When Dr. Heddiger came in to talk about a C-section, he said, "You know that I have concerns about Simon's condition." I responded, "We have only hope. We've put this in God's hands." We agreed with Dr Heddiger that Simon needn't work any harder than he had to during delivery. Within 20-30 minutes, we were in the operating room for a C-section delivery.

On September 7, 2010, at 5:40 p.m. Simon Dominic Crosier entered this world. We heard Simon's cry. He was pink, just like Melanie Ward had predicted. Dr. Heddiger said, "He's small and has the little cleft." That was fine with us. We were simply filled with joy — yet scared. A neonatologist examined him and said, "He looks good, and he's breathing on his own." When the nurse practitioner put Simon's head next to Scott's and mine, we felt overwhelming love for our little man. We were still hopeful that he would be healthy. He was perfect and so sweet!

Scott went with Simon and the doctor to the second-floor NICU. I was taken to recovery until the effects of anesthesia wore off and feeling returned to my legs and feet. When they arrived in the NICU, Scott was told to wait outside Simon's room in the Giraffe pod. The doctor told him that there were some concerns. Scott could only answer solemnly, "I know." My husband continued to pray that Simon would be fine. After they gave me the green light, I was finally wheeled to the NICU to "love on" my precious baby boy, Simon Dominic Crosier.

The next day, doctors performed an echocardiogram on Simon. Another cardiologist from Dr. Zandra's office came to Simon's room to share the findings. Dr. Bloomberg* said that Simon had a large hole in his heart, a VSD (ventricular septal defect). He also had a coarctation (a narrowing of the heart's aorta) and a PDA (patent ductus arteriosus — a persistent opening between two major blood vessels leading from the heart). I told the doctor that they had the wrong baby! This baby had experienced two fetal echocardiograms conducted by two of the most well respected pediatric cardiologists in St. Louis. Dr. Bloomberg informed us that the coarctation sometimes masks the VSD in a fetal echocardiogram. Caregivers then started an IV of prostaglandins to keep the PDA open. Typically, this drug is used to keep the PDA open while the patient awaits surgery. If Simon's PDA closed, he could die. We were sick to hear this news. Our precious Simon would need surgery for his heart now.

On Simon's third day of life, we received the news about Simon's karyotype from the FISH (fluorescence in situ hybridization) test he had received soon after his delivery. We expected the results back in the late afternoon so we were just hanging out with Simon in his room praying for his heart and healthy test results. Then Dr. Ring*, the neonatologist on staff, walked in about 1 p.m.

Dr. Ring was very candid — almost matter-of-fact — with the news. She said, "Simon has full Trisomy 18."

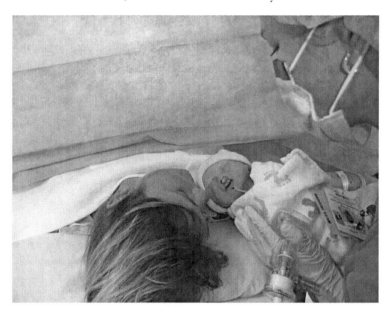

We had prayed every night for a healthy baby with the correct number of chromosomes. But now our baby had Trisomy 18, and we wondered, "Why God?" We had already lost six babies. We chose not to have an amniocentesis because we would never forgive ourselves if something happened to this human life as a result of the invasive procedure. During my pregnancy, we agreed that if our baby had Trisomy 18 we would never terminate. We loved Simon so much and hoped that he would stay with us here on earth for a while before going to heaven.

We prayed the Lord would give us the maximum time with him. At this point, Simon's cleft lip wasn't an issue. Caregivers fed him only TPN (total parenteral nutrition) through an IV. I was pumping breast milk, but they wouldn't use it to feed Simon. Maybe we could give Simon drops of breast milk through a syringe. Then we could freeze the rest because I believed and hoped the day would come when he could use it. Simon's doctors agreed.

The hospital offered us photography free of charge for family pictures. We're so glad we accepted this offer since we didn't know how long we would have Simon. I couldn't help thinking: "Do the doctors think he is going to die soon?"

I was already shaking as I went back to my room on the fifth floor at the thought of a family picture. As I was getting ready for the photograph, a medical assistant came in to take my vitals. I remember that it seemed somehow absurd to be taking my vitals when Simon's condition was of such concern. "My baby has Trisomy 18," I said. She responded, "I know, I know." I looked at her and said, "No you don't know how it feels that my baby is going to die. Please get out — just leave!"

The photographer was very nice and took several pictures with our family of five. In some photos, Scott and I held Simon, and in others, our three sons were photographed together. His caregivers were nice enough to remove Simon's oxygen mask for the pictures.

Samuel and Sean were so excited to see their baby brother. It was the first day they held Simon. Simon's nurse watched him very closely. She put a pillow under him and showed the boys how to hold him in a secure and comforting position. Samuel and Sean were so grateful to be hugging and kissing their baby brother's beautiful soft, wrinkled skin. Oh, they were so excited to hold Simon! He was finally in their arms. Samuel commented, "See, I told you he would be born and come out of your tummy." To Samuel, "Out of the tummy" meant everything was okay. He remembered that Sophia, his baby sister, died in Mommy's tummy.

We wondered how to break the diagnosis to Samuel and Sean about their long-awaited little baby brother. The doctors thought the boys should know as soon as possible. I didn't agree. Our boys prayed over my belly every night. Why rob them of the joy of their brother's company so quickly? We wanted Samuel and Sean to enjoy Simon for as long as God let us care for him. Ultimately, Scott agreed with the doctors that we should tell our boys sooner than later. We kept it simple. Simon's heart was broken and the doctors might not be able to fix it.

Simon's heart was broken and so was ours. We requested a meeting with Dr. Zandra. He conducted the second echocardiogram. Dr. Zandra explained surgery to us and that the surgeon would go through Simon's back instead of his chest. There are only a few pediatric cardiac surgeons in the area, and Dr. Andrew Fiore at Cardinal Glennon Children's Medical Center would most likely be more willing to intervene in this case. As a Catholic, prolife hospital, this institution was more likely to advocate for Simon — we hoped. Dr. Zandra informed us that many surgeons wouldn't work on a Trisomy 18 baby. He put it this way: *"The majority of pediatric heart surgeons in this area resist operating on children with Trisomy 18 or related chromosomal abnormalities. They'll cite median survival rates that are in the three to four month range. The real reason is that they believe that child is going to die and there is nothing they can do about that reality. They believe surgery on a child who is certainly going to die is not an appropriate use of resources."*

We were shocked! First we heard that during labor a Trisomy 18 baby is not even routinely monitored for heart activity. Then we learned there are only a few pediatric cardiac surgeons who will operate on a Trisomy 18 child. We wanted Simon to have every opportunity to live. We responded to Dr. Zandra that we considered Simon's time here on Earth precious and valuable no matter how long or short. To our delight and great comfort, he concurred. "I agree with Dr. Fiore, a man of great faith, that it's not up to me to decide who lives or dies," Dr. Zandra said. "I'm not empowered to make that decision. These hard medical choices should be up to the parents and God's will."

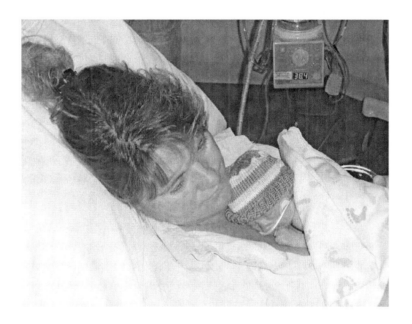

We scheduled Simon to be transported on Monday morning to Cardinal Glennon Children's Medical Center to have Dr. Fiore fix his heart. Scott and I saw Simon's case as no different than our other sons. If Samuel or Sean needed surgery, we wouldn't deny them.

I'll never forget that Sunday night. Dr. Orwell*, another neonatologist, came in to ask if we had any questions before

Simon's morning transport. I asked if the ambulance ride would stress our little boy and if I could ride with him.

Dr Orwell was very candid, explaining that I wouldn't be able to ride with Simon in the ambulance. She added that heart surgery would be dangerous for our vulnerable little boy. Sitting down with Scott and I, she answered our questions and shared information we hadn't heard from anyone else on the medical team about Simon's odds of surviving heart surgery. When she described the process of intubating him and opening up his tiny chest, we questioned ourselves, and the likelihood that little Simon would even make it off the operating table. When we asked this physician and mother sitting in front of us if she would allow her own child to endure heart surgery under these circumstances, she solemnly replied, "No."

Dr. Orwell continued to explain about the narcotics Simon would be given after the surgery. Eventually, he would have to be weaned off them. Would caregivers be able to intubate him because of Trisomy 18 and apnea? If they were not able to extubate him (get him breathing on his own), would he be on a ventilator? The doctor said he might never be able to come off the ventilator. Then, we would have another decision to make. Would we need to pull the plug? We could never do that! Maybe he would come around, but what if he couldn't? There were also many more surgeries that might follow his heart operation, such as his cleft lip procedure down the road.

We wanted to take one event at a time. We hoped everything would go well with the heart surgery. But, what if it didn't? We could lose our beautiful little 3-pound, 12-ounce Simon on the operating table. Even though he was born at 4 pounds 3 ounces, he lost weight, as most infants do initially. We would have to live with our decisions for the rest of our lives. The medical staff could walk out the hospital doors and go home to be with their families and forget about the Crosiers and Simon, our very precious child of God. Unless you truly feel it first-hand, you don't know what a burden this decision-making responsibility can be. You can only ask the Holy Spirit to touch you.

In the Giraffe pod, Simon had some medical situations. He was on humidified oxygen because of his pulmonary hypertension, complicated by his heart condition. His lungs looked fine, though. Before this he received continuous positive airway pressure for a short time. We decided not to have a circumcision performed. Simon needed to retain all his energy and stamina. He didn't have many reserves because of his heart condition. For a short time, he also was treated with bilirubin lights for jaundice. Scott always referred to this as "Simon's Sands Resort." Scott researched online and found St. Simon's Island, a resort in Georgia. We hoped to go there someday.

I wasn't able to stay overnight with Simon in the NICU because my room was on the fifth floor, due to the C-section. Simon was on the second floor. Instead, Scott would wheel me down to see Simon. After my discharge on day five, I was

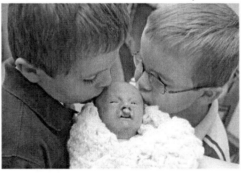

finally able to spend the night in Simon's room, relieving Scott who had stayed with Simon continually since his birth. During that time, Scott stayed on the couch next to Simon's isolette.

He sometimes heard alarms in the middle of the night, but the nurses told him not to worry. Because of breathing difficulties, Simon was put on a machine to assist his breathing through continuous positive airway pressure.

After talking with Dr. Orwell, we made the excruciating decision that night not to leave the St. Paul's NICU. Our original plan was to have the surgery at Cardinal Glennon and then be transferred back to St. Paul's if Simon still needed to be in the hospital. We kept praying that he would just be able to go home with us. We decided to stay put. We were praying that our son would be one of those Trisomy 18 children who survived until at least one-year-old. After all, each Trisomy 18 baby is unique. We asked the Lord to give us just one year with Simon.

Late that night we were transferred to a larger room that was much quieter and had a window. As we followed Simon's nurse, Sandy, I said to Scott "I feel like we're watching a movie and we're in it." We were following our precious little man with the most beautiful name in the world, Simon Dominic Crosier, to what would become our home away from home — Koala 2264.

CHAPTER FIVE

Home away from home

"As you know, the lifespan in individuals with Trisomy 18 is shortened. About 5-10 percent of babies with Trisomy 18 will live beyond one year." — letter from genetic counselor

We would provide comfort care for our baby, while pursuing every medical alternative possible. We didn't ever want Simon to suffer. We accompanied Simon to his new, much bigger home at Koala 2264. When we walked into Koala 2264 through the double glass sliding doors, to the left were the sink and cabinets where personal items, like Simon's bath accessories and bottles, could be stored. Next were the trash, soiled-linen area and supply cabinets. Above the supply cabinet hung the beautiful quilt from Grandma Lois made just for Simon. Within easy reach was the nurses' computer station to chart Simon's vitals and medical notes. To the left was Simon's crib, with monitors over it. They continually spelled out in digital detail Simon's ongoing struggle for life.

On the ledge, above his crib, was his feeding pump and an extra blank monitor. Alongside him were his oxygen and bag and mask. There was also a pastel animal curtain. I focused on the giraffe and the koala since Simon was in both of those pods. On the eastern wall was a window where the sun bathed our Simon's room in light in the morning.

There was also a bookcase with shelves where I would store photo albums, "thank-you" cards, a Praise book from my church deacon and Max Lucado's book *Fearless*. Also in the room were two couches, one blue and one green, that folded down into beds so that both my husband and I could stay overnight with Simon. Grandma stayed overnight with Simon's big brothers at home.

We used white sheets and blue blankets from the pediatric floor. I planned to get a nice blanket to match his room. To the right of the large window with white shutters there were coat hooks where we hung a clean shirt for each of the boys to change into before they held Simon. Two button-down shirts — one for me and one for Scott — were ready to wear when we kangarooed Simon. Kangaroo care involved holding our baby skin to skin on our chests so he could feel our heartbeats. Also available were a brown rocking chair and green recliner where we would spend time holding Simon. The sliding glass doors offered privacy. The sink where I could wash my face and brush my teeth in the morning was convenient. The setup of Koala 2264 was efficient. But God's timing was perfect — the room had been built just a few months prior to Simon's arrival.

Shortly after Simon began his stay in the Koala pod, the genetic counselor dropped off an envelope with "Simon Crosier" written on the front. The letter was written on September 10, 2010. Chris came into Simon's room in the Giraffe pod after we received the Trisomy 18 diagnosis. I didn't remember what she looked like, and I barely remember her being in his room. We were so upset about our little guy.

The letter started off very nicely. It basically said, "Congratulations on the birth of your son Simon. It went on to describe Trisomy 18. "Having an extra copy of a chromosome is caused by a pair of chromosomes failing to split into two different cells during the egg or sperm formation," the letter said. "It's important to know that there is nothing that a parent does before or during a pregnancy to cause Trisomy 18. "

The letter also said that Simon had a complex heart defect. It also said, "As you know, the lifespan in individuals with Trisomy 18 is shortened. About 5-10 percent of babies with Trisomy 18 will live beyond one year. There are children with Trisomy 18 who have lived longer than five years. Children with Trisomy 18 who survive beyond infancy can advance in their developmental skills although their development is very much delayed. A child with Trisomy 18 will recognize family members and other loved ones and interact with them." We prayed and hoped that Simon would live beyond infancy.

We also continued to do research beyond the information contained in the letter. Our findings concluded that about 90 percent of Trisomy 18 children have heart defects. Simon had been diagnosed with a VSD (Ventricular Septal Defect) and a coarctation. Trisomy 18 children also may have a persisting normal PDA (Patent Ductus Arteriosus) that might contribute to increased difficulty in breathing or feeding. They may also have persistent increased pulmonary vascular resistance, often referred to as pulmonary hypertension. Research indicates that the more severe the heart abnormalities are the more likely early death is from cardiopulmonary disease or congestive heart failure. These infants often have difficulty gaining weight because of their heart problems. Simon's heart was very damaged. Oh, how we prayed that God, the Great Physician, would just fix it!

We were learning that babies with Trisomy 18 require special care and constant attention. Caring for the child and paying attention for any signs of infection, illness and heart problems required meetings with the medical team on a regular basis. Our goal was to stay on top of Simon's conditions and look for problems before issues came up.

*Lola, Simon's nurse, suggested we start a Caring Bridge site online. Most of our doctors and nurses were so kind and loving that we decided to look into it. Staci, Scott's sister, set up Simon's Caring Bridge site and uploaded pictures. This became our connection with our community outside the hospital and a way to update everyone on Simon. Our community supporters' postings gave us strength and hope to get through each day. Those who posted offered their love, prayers and support in a very real way even if it was online. We frequently updated Simon's status on the Caring Bridge journal we began. Many Caring Bridge people became Simon's biggest fans.

Here are just a few of the hundreds of postings that meant so much to our family, and Simon.

- **Saturday, September 11, 2010, 3:21 p.m.**

  Simon, You don't know me, but I know YOU. You were blessed to have Angels who love you enough to bring you into this wonderful family. I know you are being shown more love than some babies will ever know in a lifetime. I pray for you all the time. You are a sweetheart and I love you so much.

  Betty Schwant

  Monday, September 13, 2010, 11:54 a.m.

  To Sheryl, Scott and boys-my heart has been sooo heavy for you. You have no idea how many people are praying for you all. Simon is our little blessing from God. A huge cyber hug to you, much love and will continue to storm the heavens with prayers

  -Love you-
  Mary McEvoy

- **Monday, September 13, 2010, 12:33 p.m.**

  Words can't express my heartfelt emotion. God has
  given a special gift to all of us. Simon has done
  powerful things for many even before he was born.
  May the love and strength from God give guidance
  and comfort to the Crosier family. May you find a
  peace from all the love.
  I continue to offer prayers for you.
  God bless!
  Jo Berlinger

- **Monday, September 13, 2010, 4:30 p.m.**

  Dear Crosiers: I am praying for you and baby Simon
  and you are in my thoughts all the time. I pray that
  Simon will be, like his namesake Simon Peter, a
  "rock" for your faith and love. I know Our Lord
  holds Simon very close, and your faith is beautiful to
  see. My heart goes out to you all!!!
  With love and prayers and every good thought
  Susan Fitzpatrick

- **Wednesday, September 15, 2010, 12:26 p.m.**

  Dear Simon,

  Welcome to this wacky, wonderful world! Already
  you have brought such tremendous love and joy to
  your family, and you have taught hundreds of praying
  people such lessons of faith, courage and trust. Thank
  you!

You continue to be in my heart and prayers along with your mommy, daddy and brothers. Peace to you all.

Love,
Kate Boemeke Uptergrove

- **Wednesday, September 15, 2010, 8:45 a.m.**

Just a note to let you know I'm thinking and praying for the whole family. I don't know the family, but work at the same company as the father. I heard the family's story through coworkers.

I had a daughter with Trisomy 18 born 02/03/1992 (Kathrylyn Tyler). Unfortunately, four days later she passed away. I loved every moment I was able to spend with her.

There have been so many advancements in medicine over the past 18 years! Take care and may God bless you all with many blessings!

Paula Kehrer

- **Wednesday, September 15, 2010, 2:04 p.m.**

Dear Sheryl - Please know that you and your family are in our thoughts and prayers. Simon is such a tiny person but touches many lives because he reminds us all that each day is to be treasured and we should embrace the life & gifts we've been given. May each day with him be a blessing and his precious love give you the strength you need. We're sending you and your family a big electronic hug.

Emily, Ian & Oliver Hornstra

- **Friday, September 17, 2010 10:34 AM**

Dear Ms. Sheryl,

Last night I read some of the messages you have been receiving, and I woke up this morning thinking about your journey. My first thoughts were about how you have shown "Our Saturday Night Live Group" how the Living Bible works. You have been teaching us right along. I opened the Bible and read the passage **eyes have not seen, ears have not heard.** I stopped and thought, "Oh yes, I have been honored to watch right before my eyes **Faith, Hope and Love** in action. We are all blessed to see love around us. But watching the depth of this Faith and Hope is God's gift for the taking. Thank you.

To You, your family and baby Simon the prayers will continue as you journey with the Lord. Lots of Love, Renee Quackenbush

- **Thursday, November 11, 2010, 4:54 p.m.**

Simon, my dear little Simon - In the early hour of this new day, while all around me was asleep, I realized that after being a part of your world for four days, I would not be seeing you. Then I felt a tap, tap, tap in my heart, and there you were reminding me that you, in your silence and in your sweet spirit, are not that far away after all.

The enriching experience I was so blessed to have with you, your family and the wonderful caring professionals was an intense and absorbing kind of love that only the power of God could create. So many gifts surround you.

I remembered that it was a man named Simon who carried the cross for Jesus. Through thousands of prayers we know Jesus is now carrying you, Simon, through these recent days of blessed peaceful sleep and restful hours. God's angels are keeping you safe.

Simon, your name is written across many hearts across the miles. It means, "to be heard." We like that.

I love you. Auntie J

Judy Ford

- **Thursday, November 25, 2010, 10:06 p.m.**

Thank you, Simon, for teaching me that life is indeed a gift, that each moment is a blessing from God, and that God's plans are always better than my own. I thank God for your family, who continue to teach me the importance of faith, hope, trust and confidence in a God who is always there, even when it is difficult to find Him. May each of you continue to draw strength from each other, and from the God, who made this all possible.

Sister Chris De Anna

CHAPTER SIX

The fight of a lifetime

"She walked me over to your bed and there you were — the most beautiful baby I had ever seen! You were so incredibly perfect in every way." — Lisa, family friend

One week later, we learned that Simon's condition had weakened. We decided not to expose his vulnerable body to heart surgery. It was time to put in a PICC (peripherally inserted central catheter) line to infuse his prostaglandins. Prostaglandins are fatty acid components of cell membranes that have proven, in clinical studies with newborns suffering heart defects, to play a crucial role in keeping these babies alive. The medication allows a specialized fetal blood vessel (the ductus arteriosus) to remain open, allowing sufficient oxygenation of the infant's blood for survival. The medical staff suggested taking the IV line out of Simon's umbilical cord and moving it to his foot. This placement reduced the chance for infection and made it easier to dress Simon. The line change went smoothly. Simon's nurse *Pam was beside him feeding him sucrose and my breast milk.

After the doctors placed the PICC line, they started feeding Simon his breast milk through a tube that went in his nose and then down into his stomach. Previously, he received his milk from a syringe. That made his Mommy and Daddy very happy. Simon was a fighter! He continued to fight for his life.

Our primary concern was central apnea, which is a periodic interruption of breathing. Obstructive apnea could also account for breathing difficulties, but might be easier for doctors to treat. Fortunately, at this point, his apnea episodes were infrequent.

We were really finding out what living in the moment means. We cherished every second with Simon because he was teaching us all lessons in love and hope. I must admit, our joy was attacked each time we were given details of how he might pass. Well-meaning people advised us to plan his funeral. The constant negativity was stressful — medical professionals were telling us we could lose him at any time. Our unconditional love and Simon's presence kept us going. Yes, we challenged everything we were told because we wanted the best for our little man. We knew that Simon was quietly, in his own way, making us even more compassionate human beings. Simon's courageous struggle was molding us into the people we knew we could be.

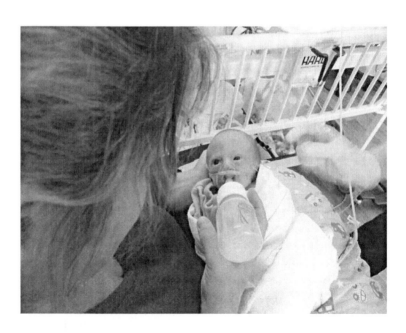

Simon devoured the breast milk. By 1½ weeks of age, he tolerated 1½ tsp. every three hours. We dressed Simon in preemie clothes, and he loved being swaddled in his blanket. That was good news because prior to the PICC line, it was impossible to wrap him up in that way. There were other positives, too. He no longer needed the incubator to keep him warm. He was doing well in his crib. He was breathing on his own with very little support, although he continued to receive humidified oxygen.

We continued to give Simon drops of breast milk in the syringe. Big brothers enjoyed sharing in this loving task. They knew they were feeding Simon and helping to keep him alive. I remained hopeful that one day the boys could give him a bottle. His nurse Lola gave him sucrose or breast milk while the transport nurse performed a test or a procedure. As Simon lay there, helpless and so vulnerable, I again felt anxious and shaken to my core. At our request, the nurses gave Simon breast milk through a feeding tube. He tolerated his feedings very well.

Lola became a very trusted and loved member of Simon's nursing team. She described one of her early meetings with him this way:

"It was a sunny September morning. The warm sun filled Simon's little corner room in the Koala Pod. A new day was about to begin in room 64. As I came in to say 'good morning' to my new friend Simon, I noticed his sweet little eyes peeking up at me. He was wide awake! His little eyebrows arched upward as though he was expecting something to happen. He was ready to meet the day! Mom was getting comfortable in the recliner next to his crib and preparing for some very special Kangaroo time with Simon. Kangaroo time is a very special time when moms and dads hold their naked little babies up against their hearts as they snuggle together under a nice warm blanket. For most babies and parents, this is their favorite time of day! Because Simon was extra special, he got all the Kangaroo time he wanted."

Another one of Simon's nurses, Sandy*, asked me, "Do you have clothes for him?" I thought they were suggesting we take more family pictures because they kept talking about enjoying every moment. We didn't know how long we would have him. We knew that Trisomy 18 is unpredictable, and as Dr. Pang said many times, "Simon will tell us his story." He meant that Simon would tell us when he was ready to give up the fight.

We brought in little blue, green and other colored baby boy outfits. We made sure the majority of his outfits snapped up the front for easy access to his PICC line. This was the perfect time for portraits of Simon in his new clothes! Heidi Drexler Photography came in to capture Simon and his new home. Heidi, a family friend, did an amazing job. She went beyond the call of duty by creating a black and white album of her photographs of Simon. It was beautiful — even the foot pictures with the PICC line. Heidi, with her photographer's eye, looked into my little boy's eyes and touched the beauty of his spotless soul.

Heidi expressed her thoughts with these lovely words:

"I am certain that photography is a gift I have been given. I meet new families every day with children of all ages...some brand new and a few days old, some with their first lost tooth and others about to go away to college. I always feel grateful that I can give parents a piece of memory of their child at that very moment. But nothing could prepare me for what I experienced photographing Simon. From the minute I stepped foot into the hospital intensive care unit, I knew my 'job' was bigger than me. I had a responsibility. I wanted to capture Simon and his family and what life was like living in the ICU. I wanted Simon's Mom to look at these photographs and remember exactly what it was like: The smell, the nurses, the beeping of machines, the light as it pours in from the window — Simon. I wanted her to remember Simon. I wanted to give the family something to hold on to forever. Even when the memories fade and they are desperately trying to remember what it was like...they would have these photographs to bring you back. Simon was only on this earth for a

short time, but he was a fighter, a brother, a son, a patient and an angel. I will forever remember Simon and what he taught me. He taught me my gift is for a reason — and for that I'm grateful."

Another dear friend, Lisa, later wrote directly to Simon about the impact he had on her during her first visit:

"I remember the pride I felt the day your mom called to invite me to the hospital to meet you," Lisa wrote. *"It was a busy day like any other, but this one was special because of you. I walked into your room to first find your beautiful mother. She walked me over to your bed and there you were —the most beautiful baby I had ever seen! You were so incredibly perfect in every way. I felt like I knew you long before that moment because your mother and I would talk excitedly anticipating your arrival when you were still in her belly. I felt so honored and privileged to be in your presence. You slept for most of my visit, but you did open those big eyes for a while. You left me speechless, Simon. All I could do was stare into your eyes. Time stood still as I soaked up every second with you. I will never forget meeting you or the way you touched my heart and all of our lives."*

Simon continued to fight for his life, but his doctors seemed to believe it would be a short struggle. They told us that with any infusion line, there is always a chance for infection. But, we thought it was far too soon for the doctors to talk to us about removing the prostaglandins. We wondered why, at that point, they were now saying we needed to worry about infection. It was frightening to think that a blood infection like sepsis could take Simon away so quickly.

The doctors asked us how we wanted them to treat Simon if he developed an infection. Well, how would you treat any infection? Of course — with an antibiotic! They sometimes looked at us as if we were crazy. They pointed out we would have to put in an IV, which would not be comfortable for Simon. We were thinking if the IV was needed to save him, little Simon could endure the stick.

My husband, a man who has never been afraid to speak his mind, had his own forceful Simon statement that he often repeated to Simon's medical team when he became impatient with their negativity.

"We will not do anything to expedite his demise," he said. Scott grew up in a rural Kansas town where everyday life meant taking care of your neighbor. His no-nonsense upbringing blends with his accountants training to leave little room in his steadfast personality for imprecise communication. "We just wanted the facts about Simon's condition delivered with a bit of compassion," Scott explained. "Some of the people caring for my son exemplified the best kindness and sensitivity you hope for in medical professionals, or any human being. But in too many instances, his doctors conveyed the impression that Simon's condition made him less of a priority for their time. Certainly less of a candidate for the same procedures they might have tried with an infant with the same heart problems, but without Edwards syndrome, otherwise known as Trisomy 18."

Scott was right! Simon was not a syndrome. He was our beautiful son and a child of God. I protected him from the moment of conception and would do so throughout his time here on earth. We wanted Simon to only know love. He will always be a part of our family.

We continued to pray that Simon wouldn't get an infection. But we backed up our constant prayers with our own research. We looked into the long-term use of prostaglandins. We searched online and found a boy who was on this medication for more than 200 days. Again we wondered why doctors seemed anxious to get Simon off the prostaglandins? Was it because Simon had Trisomy 18?

So the conversations about prostaglandins continued. One of Simon's nurses commented that she couldn't believe they put Simon on this medication. She said they don't usually put a baby with Trisomy 18 on prostaglandins. We were appalled to think caregivers would deny these babies treatment. This was extremely upsetting to me. I decided to ask one of the neonatologists, Dr. Orwell if this was true. She said they would have treated Simon this way even if they knew he had Trisomy 18. Still, I couldn't help but wonder about other babies who shared Simon's condition or other life-threatening challenges.

Every night the boys told Simon goodnight on the phone. Sean would say, "No pillow fights with Mommy. I love you Simon." And Samuel would say, "Goodnight Simon. I love you — you are my best buddy." Simon listened so closely and smiled. I could tell he was saying, "I love you big brothers."

The hospital even set up a Webcam in Simon's room so his big brothers could watch him at night from home. Unfortunately Samuel and Sean soon refused to go to bed at night because they were so engrossed in "looking out" for Simon. We had to turn it off at a set time to make sure Simon's caring brothers wouldn't stay up too late and fall asleep at their school desks the next morning.

CHAPTER SEVEN

Promise keepers

Simon would let us know what he wanted to hear. One night Mary tried to change his CDs. He opened his eyes and looked at her raising his contractured (crooked) index finger and made himself heard.

Scott always keeps his promises. He bought Samuel and Sean a bunk bed. He had their room painted in NASCAR style. The boys also wanted one wall with only St. Louis sports stuff, including the Cardinals, Rams and Blues. They were waiting for their baby brother to come home to sleep in the bedroom next to theirs, which was Sean's old bedroom. Sean would talk about having Simon lay in the bunk bed with them. After all, Simon was already one of "the boys."

We never lost hope that someday, Simon could come home. But, for that time, Koala 2264 was his home and ours, too. We received comforting gifts and purchased some very soft warm blankets. Our favorite was from our friend, Maureen. It's light blue with our son's name and date of birth. His blankets came in handy when we held him tight, Kangarooed him or gave him a massage, which was a relaxation technique that Simon's physical therapists taught us. There were times he was so relaxed. I could massage him endlessly. He looked me in the eyes as I massaged his arms, hands and legs. These days were perfect. We hoped for many more.

We made Simon's room a home away from home for the boys. Sean and Samuel were able to have a sleepover. We watched Mary Poppins on TV, and Simon loved the music. It was so nice to be together as a family. Our adorable little boy looked around to find out where the music was coming from. Samuel loved to sing "*Supercalifragilisticexpialidocious*" to his baby brother. We kept thinking and wondering if Simon would ever come to our home and see the TV in our living room?

One night during the first month of Simon's stay at St. Paul's, we met Mary*, a very pretty Indian woman. Mary worked the weekend with Simon, so even his big brothers got to know her. They had plenty of questions for Mary about India. They wanted to know all about king cobras and monkeys. Mary later brought in several books on reptiles and snakes native to India. These books became part of their library in Simon's room in the Koala pod.

Following is a note that Mary wrote to us on Simon's behalf that first weekend she cared for him. On it was a picture of Simon and a trophy saying, #1 Fan.

To My Dear Mom and Dad,
I think it is important for you to know how much I love you both
I know in my heart that you have both worked so hard for me
I bask in the luxury of love, faith and hope.
The quick smile at my silliness, the glistening of your eyes due to my trial and tribulations and the pitter patter of your heart
When you worry about me, it has not gone unnoticed.
As I grow strong every day, I do hope I lessen your sorrow.
I am trying very hard to stay out of mischief
I would like to award you with this certificate in recognition of your dedication to me.

Love you always
Your dear sweet Simon

Unfortunately, our next night nurse, Tracey* presented a different situation. This particular night both Grandma Lois and I spent a great deal of time walking the halls trying to find her. The nurse covering for Tracey said she was pumping breast milk. Tracey had a baby at home that she needed to pump for. At least three times that night we asked about our night nurse's location and received the same answer. She was pumping.

We were increasingly upset because Simon's oxygen saturation levels dropped frequently. One morning at 6 a.m. we pushed the call button for Tracey. I noticed her slowly walking down the hall with her bag holding her breast pump items. I told her, "You have four healthy children at home and my son is terminal, I expect you to be attentive to his needs when you are here." Tracey said the nurse who was covering for her should have been more attentive. I talked to the nursing supervisor and insisted that Simon never have Tracey again. The nursing supervisor complied with our wishes immediately. I still think about the possible consequences if Grandma Lois and I were not there that night to ensure someone was always in the room with Simon.

On Sept. 20 Simon's complete medical team met face-to-face to assess him and determine next steps with his care. The next day doctors reduced his dose of prostaglandin by half. The expectation was that the smaller dose wouldn't reduce the medicine's effectiveness in keeping his heart duct open, but it might help reduce Simon's apnea episodes. We tried to build some normal routine into our days as Samuel and Sean came to visit Simon each day after school. Grandma Lois was so helpful getting the boys to and from school and being their limo service to the hospital.

The family lounge became very familiar to Samuel and Sean. After holding Simon, they enjoyed a snack and a juice box or milk in the family lounge. We even maintained a personal space in the cabinet that stored our family snacks. We stored some dinners in the refrigerator. When Simon was having difficulty breathing, one of us would take the boys down the hall to the lounge. We established a code with some of his nurses when it was time for the boys to leave the room. Scott and I didn't want the boys to see their brother struggling to breathe or hear the alarms sounding.

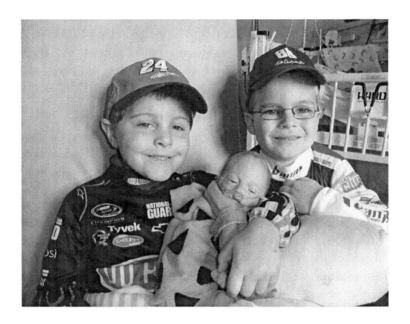

Big brothers Samuel and Sean had a routine for visiting their baby brother. After school they came to the hospital, ran up the walkway to the yellow elevators, pushed "2" and signed their names at the front desk. At that point, they got a visitor sticker reflecting the color of the day. "Big" and "Bigger" Brother was written on their stickers. They made bets with each other to see who knew the right color. They loved to talk with the staff while they were signing in about NASCAR. Everyone knew Samuel was a Jeff Gordon fan and Sean was a fan of Dale Earnhardt Jr. After the automatic doors opened, they immediately went to the large sinks and soaped up thoroughly. They never wanted Simon to catch bad germs. As they entered the room, they would usually be loud and excited. Often, we had to calm them down. They anxiously changed into their clean t-shirts hanging in Simon's room. They waited as patiently as they could to hold their little brother.

On the morning of September 23, Simon had a few more serious apnea episodes. He continued to show great resiliency and had had a less eventful and more relaxing afternoon. He spent most of the day kangarooing with Mommy and Daddy and eagerly awaited the arrival of his big brothers after school.

Samuel and Sean wore their Simon shirts with pride. Scott's sisters Auntie Staci and Auntie Laurie had all three brothers' pictures placed on the shirts. Both said, "Simon's big brother." On the back of each shirt were the boys' names.

Another shirt for each boy was produced with the compassionate assistance of nurse Mary. One night, Mary brought in an orange and a blue t -shirt with paints. Mary later explained to me that her connection to Simon was immediate and based on spiritual hope, not the pessimism of a challenging diagnosis. *"The atmosphere with some of my colleagues walking into Simon's room was like walking into a funeral, like his death already happened,"* she remembered. *"Because of his heart rate and oxygen saturation rates, they acted as if there was not much hope, nothing further they could do. But the child's eyes opened and I looked into his eyes and I told myself, Simon doesn't need this atmosphere. Give him what he deserves. He was like Prince Charming to me."*

Mary always called Simon her Prince Charming. Addressing Simon as King or Prince was a frequent occurrence. On the dry-erase board in the Koala pod, Mary drew a picture and wrote "Simon's Castle." Each wonderful gesture of this faith-filled woman didn't go unnoticed by Simon or his parents.

"My sense of faith has carried me through life," Mary told me. *"I connected with Simon through my heart and not as a medical case. He drew me to him with silent eyes."*

Mary could read Simon's moods like no one else on the nursing staff. *"Simon made fussy noises,"* she said. *"If he didn't like certain music, he would let you know. At night he stayed awake and interacted with me with his unique personality. Sometimes, if he was angry, he wouldn't look at me, but usually he looked at me clearly. He had a hooked finger, and he hooked everyone's heart."*

Grandma Lois and I did our part to lighten the atmosphere in Simon's room. And the boys were wildly excited to smash their hands in the fabric paint to mold their own handprint. We decided to do Simon's footprints instead. In his room, Simon was king. He was so cooperative and patient. He had so many fine qualities, if only we all could be like him. Katrina, his PICC line nurse, Pam, his primary nurse, and I worked together to put his footprints on both the eight plates and the big brothers' t-shirts. Little did Simon know his footprints were being made with all the love and spirit that captured his personality and would be a forever keepsake.

Each day we experienced more ups and downs, and September 25 was no different. We met with Simon's doctor, and he said that Simon looked good and was holding his own. Simon was now looking for his feedings 20-30 minutes early. This was a good sign that could lead to another increase in feeding quantity.

Auntie Laurie and Auntie Staci, Scott's sisters, came in from Kansas to meet their precious little nephew. They made sure they got lots of pictures and told Simon how they had been waiting to meet him and how much they loved him. They both shed tears of joy. They simply fell in love with him very quickly. The aunties also did a great job entertaining Simon's big brothers. They took them wherever they wanted to go. Samuel and Sean had a ball!

A quick trip to Kohl's was needed. I purchased a soft light blue blanket and a navy blue fleece blanket. I was looking forward to having soft, warm things for my warm baby. These items made Simon's room even more of a home. Some nights I sobbed and shook in my pillow, always wanting Simon to be here, even if it had to be in a hospital room.

Simon continued to hold his own and September 28 was his 21st wonderful day. He continued to amaze us with his strength and toughness. His feedings continued at 28 ml every three hours. He knew when it was time to eat. He also got more active with his arm and leg movements, so we cherished each wonderful improvement. Many of his nurses commented on how well he interacted with us and his environment.

Catherine*, one of Simon's night nurses, brought in a couple of CDs we'll always cherish, including Disney lullabies, which we played all day and night. Some of the other music we played was baby Bible songs, rainforest nature's lullabies, Susan Boyle's "the gift," and soft, relaxing music from our friend Sheila that had enjoyed all during my pregnancy. Simon loved his music and his room was calm and peaceful.

Whatever we could do to make life enjoyable and entertaining for Simon, we did. One day I remember sending Grandma Lois out to buy a mobile. She asked, "Today?" I said "Yes, we would like to have one today because Simon is King!" Grandma Lois went to *Babies r Us* and bought Simon a mobile. Our little King loved to watch the animals spin and listened to the music. Simon also enjoyed an orange-and-black-striped tiger from Sean and a blue bear from Samuel. The bear was a balloon animal that Samuel's second-grade class gave him along with cards that each of Samuel's classmates made. Sean's kindergarten classmates also made cards for Simon.

Simon's relaxation time included bath time. All of his cords were off, and he was finally free. Simon would also humor us as well. During his first tub bath, he pooped in the water. Big brothers really got a kick out of this. Not only did Simon poop in his bathtub, he peed on Mommy and his nurses. Sean loved to share these stories with his kindergarten class.

Asking his teacher Mrs. Boone if it was okay to tell, she responded, "Go right ahead."

Bath time was so special. He would watch us, relax and close his eyes. He loved the boys using the washcloths to clean him and pour warm water over him with little bottles. He also liked to have baby lotion gently rubbed on him. Then, we'd put him in a soft fuzzy outfit to wear. So comfy!

Simon also loved to nurse for comfort. Lola, his nurse, captures one of those unforgettable moments: "This particular morning Simon was extra spunky," Lola recalled:

"As he settled on his Mom's chest, he kept rooting around looking for something to eat! This really surprised me because, up to this point, Simon was working hard to breathe and keeping his heart pumping. He hadn't shown an interest in eating. Those of us who loved Simon were eager to give him the things he wanted. So after asking permission from the doctor, I suggested that mom allow Simon to breastfeed. Mom was supplying pumped breast milk for Simon's tube feedings. That day, Simon was feeling hungry, and he was looking for his food. This time it wasn't coming from a tube. It was coming from his Mom! It was so good to see that strength in him. It was one of many days that filled us with a glimmer of hope. There was not a dry eye in Simon's room that day. It was such a joy to see him nuzzling around looking for his food and finding exactly what he wanted."

He couldn't breast feed on a regular basis because we couldn't monitor the amount of milk he was getting. But he loved the bottle of breast milk, and that way we could have his speech therapist come in to listen to him swallow. He was very coordinated. We didn't want him to use up too much energy in the effort of feeding. We didn't want him working too hard because of his poor little heart.

We had great hope. He was alive! That hopeless statement, "incompatible with life," is so heart-piercing. Simon was with us and we were proud parents. Do we really know how long any of our children will live? Life has no guarantees. It's a mystery, just like death. Simon was not incompatible with life. After all, the doctors didn't think he would make it past the first week. He was still with us and was our gift from God. Our job was to provide, protect and nurture our child. We were happy being Simon's parents, and Samuel and Sean were happy being his big brothers.

After school each day, big brothers came to visit. They told Simon about their day and their experiences. They read books to him. Samuel would read "Diary of a Wimpy Kid" and reptile books. Samuel also practiced the National Anthem that he would be singing in October at the Rams game when Kirkwood Children's Chorale was invited to perform. Was Samuel nervous in front of thousands of people? No, because Samuel had practiced constantly in front of Simon. Simon loved to hear the boys sing. Just the sound of their voices was music to his ears. His big eyes would search for the source of the joyful noise.

One night Daddy read Simon, "Goodnight Moon." Scott thought, "Wow it worked." Simon closed his eyes and fell asleep. After Scott said "the end," Simon popped open his big blue eyes and wanted more. So Scott read the story again. Simon had his nights and days mixed up. He wanted to play all night with his night nurse and sleep in the day. Fortunately, this did not last too long. I needed to sleep, too.

Sleep was not an option when Simon started having apnea. Alarms went off and nurses bolted in. Simon usually recovered on his own, but, sometimes, his caregivers assisted him with his oxygen flow through a bag and mask. This was always a matter of life or death. We insisted on basic resuscitation in the form of immediate access to oxygen and assisted ventilation via air bag and mask. We could never stand by and watch him struggle for breath.

I'll never forget the time I went to use the restroom and walked into his room, only to find him lying in his crib on his side staring at me. I said, "Simon what are you doing looking at Mama that way?" He was so still and wasn't blinking. Then, the alarm sounded. It was a terrifying apnea episode. During these apnea episodes his nurse, Pam*, would try to talk us out of assisting his breathing with an air bag. She argued that the bag was uncomfortable. How would she really know? She tried to describe it as hanging out the car window with the wind blowing in your mouth.

Pam had apparently expressed her concern about caring for a baby like Simon on her first day with our son. She complained to Mary, "What am I supposed to do, he has Trisomy 18?"

Simon continued to tolerate his breast milk feedings, and the doctors gradually increased his amounts. Another harsh term used to describe Trisomy 18 is "failure to thrive." Well, Simon was growing and gaining weight. To us, any little bit of growth was awesome. Both terms, "failure to thrive" and "incompatible with life," are so harsh. They seemed unnecessary. Simon was growing and his life was valuable. With every little victory, our hope grew and we celebrated our precious son.

A few of Simon's nurses had hope for him. We certainly could tell which ones did. Those nurses were loyal to Simon, and their devotion and warmth would fill his room. For example, Lola took a stand and requested a care conference for our little guy. When she presented her views to the medical director, he said, "We don't really do care conferences for terminal kids." Lola then said, "They are the ones who need care conferences most." She believed in the need for consistency.

Every patient should have a fighting chance. We were appalled to hear the response to her request. Once again caregivers were not valuing his life. Was this because Simon had Trisomy 18? Did this doctor actually use the term "terminal kids?" Maybe he really just meant Trisomy 18? Simon was not a terminal illness or a syndrome. He was our beloved, precious son. Lola understood our frustration and later detailed her view that a comprehensive care plan was urgently needed for children like Simon.

"On my first day caring for Simon I noticed how many diverse opinions Scott and Sheryl were getting from caregivers," she recalled. "They've not gone through this situation before, their family is just beginning to deal with devastating news, and they're being bombarded with opinions from people they don't know. It's overwhelming. My heart went out to the family. How were they processing this? They were deluged with recommendations about heart and plastic surgery and feeding and respiration options. They processed endless pharmacy issues with the prostaglandins. They needed a consistent approach with all their doctors and nurses. They needed a care plan. The plan lays out how the medical team should respond. We need to all be coming from the same direction, in agreement.

"Some people thought this approach was not necessary," she added. "I guess they concluded Simon had no chance to survive, but to families like the Crosiers, each day is a gift, a blessing."

Simon had another apnea episode at 6:30 a.m. on October 1. His heart rate dropped and his blood oxygen levels became dangerously low. The great news was that he recovered on his own fairly quickly. The next couple of days and nights were good for Simon. We still constantly watched his monitor for any changes. The medical staff was always near as well.

We celebrated Sean's 6th birthday with Simon the next day. The nurses even produced a present from Simon to Sean, a soccer ball. Sean loves soccer, and Simon knew this. We went out for dinner and then had cake in the family lounge. I know Simon passed along his own birthday wishes to his big brother Sean. The day after Sean's birthday, Samuel sang the National Anthem at the Rams game. I'm sure Simon was very proud of his big brother. We're thankful for the times we were able to balance the care Simon required with the loving attention Samuel and Sean needed.

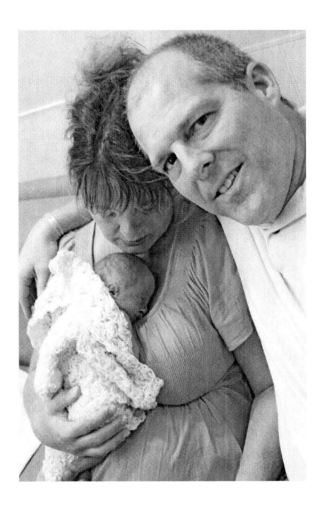

In early October, Simon continued to hold his own and actually tolerated some changes. First, his medical team changed the type of oxygen he was getting so he no longer received the humidified variety and fluid no longer got in his nose. He quickly moved from .5 liters of oxygen flow to only .1 liters. As a result, he continued to move closer to breathing completely on his own. His feedings continued to go well. He received 28mL every three hours. Simon was gaining weight at his own pace. He spent much more time awake and alert, which was nice for us because we so enjoyed interacting with him.

A special package arrived that day. Scott's sisters Auntie Staci and Auntie Laurie sent a beautiful crystal engraved frame with a picture of Daddy holding Simon. They sent me a heart locket necklace, one side displaying Simon with Scott and me; the other picturing Simon and his big brothers.

We started to celebrate Simon's monthly birthdays. I'll never forget Simon's nurse, Sandy, taking a picture of him early in the morning. He was so bright-eyed. He had his pacifier in his mouth and an adorable crinkle marked his forehead. She hung this picture with a birthday horn on the wall in the Koala pod. The adorable outfits she bought him were so sweet. He was really styling!

Simon celebrated his one-month birthday on October 7. Our son was defying all the odds. We continued to do our best to live in the moment. Unfortunately, the next day, Friday, Simon had several apnea episodes. During one, *Nancy, his nurse during the shift, said, "He is not responding." My heart sank. I asked a preoccupied housekeeper who was mopping the floor to please leave. "My baby is in terrible danger," I said. The doctor and several other nurses entered Simon's room. One of them called Scott to tell him to hurry back to the hospital. Simon did self-recover, but this time, more slowly. I asked why Nancy didn't use the oxygen mask. She said, "On his chart it says 'Do not resuscitate.'" In her opinion, that meant no bag and mask. I said, "We've authorized the bag and mask. We only said 'no' to CPR."

One of the reasons we agreed to no CPR was because time and again we were told that it could break Simon's ribs. Also, the doctors did not feel comfortable intubating Simon. In fact, one physician insisted he would not intubate him. Again, we wondered if it was just because Simon had Trisomy 18? We questioned and challenged everything. We then demanded more clarification in his chart. The doctors sent a memo to all of Simon's caregivers so this misleading "do not resuscitate" order wouldn't impact Simon's care again.

I thought of this episode much later during a conversation I had with my friend and one of the nation's top academic experts on outcomes for children with Trisomy 18, Debbie Bruns, Ph.D. She explained:

"The medical community knows certain medicine can cause a reaction, such as anti- seizure medicine. Let's say that a child like Simon codes (goes into severe cardiac arrest). Doctors are trained in this situation to administer specific types of medicine, sometimes regardless of taking into account additional factors.

"The medical team makes a recommendation on whether a child should be partially or fully tube-fed based on specific medical factors. It's crucial that one of those considerations be the adverse impact of removing this shared experience between child and parent," she added. *"Even when a child can't eat by mouth, shared experiences at the family table should be encouraged.*

"The same can be said of recommending or placing a Do Not Resuscitate (DNR) order in a chart for a child with Trisomy 18," Debbie said. *"The medical team is looking at familiar protocols, and the parents are left to battle for their child."*

Despite the occasional disagreements, most of Simon's nurses shared a deep devotion to him and were deeply affected by his spirit. One of his most attentive caregivers, Catherine, called it the "Simon Effect." She described it this way:

"Simon taught all who cared for him that we all have an assignment from God, and He has allotted a specific amount of time for each of us to accomplish that. Simon was here on a special assignment, and so he didn't need as many days as some of us do.

"Simon taught me to look deeper for a purpose in life, no matter how little the soul, or how short their stay may be. He taught me to always persist and never give up. Every person has a potential, which is only

limited by others. People will miss so much if they don't look beyond the obvious physical challenges to the way that such precious people can change their environment and the people whom they come in contact with."

Another nurse, *Wendy, added:

"When I close my eyes and think of Simon, I see a bright eyed, beautiful baby boy who came to offer us a fresh look at life. How blessed I am that little Simon's life crossed paths with mine. Perhaps that was his mission . . . to leave us with his beautiful blessings to ponder and to teach us.

What were these beautiful blessings from Simon? He showed us to treasure life and love. He gave us the gift of knowledge . . . that life, no matter how brief, and a baby, no matter how tiny, can make an impact on the world. He confirmed for us that life is fragile and that every moment counts. He taught us to soak in love, like he sweetly accepted the love given so tenderly by his wonderful family. He proved for us the need to slow down and enjoy the sweetness of one so pure from God. He blessed us with understanding that all life is beautiful end to end and encouraged us not to be afraid of living or of letting go."

October 8 was a challenging day. Simon had four apnea episodes. The doctors and nurses told us that the frequency and severity of episodes usually indicated declining health.

At that point, I was getting very nervous about the weekends. Scott started to stay with me in Simon's room on the weekends, and we asked Grandma Lois to stay with the big boys. Eventually we worked out a schedule where I stayed overnight during the week and Scott slept overnight with Simon on weekends. It was great bonding time for Daddy and Simon. It was also nice for Mommy to be with the big brothers at home.

During the week, I went home to shower every three days and then rushed back to the hospital. Fortunately, we only lived nine miles away. That day I was speeding home to shower because I was worried about Simon's hearing test. While I was away to take care of tasks like that, Grandma Lois covered for me in Simon's room for a few hours. My distraction led to me being pulled over by a police officer for speeding. I told him that Simon was in the NICU and was terminal. I also said I was trying to get home to shower quickly so I could get back to the hospital to be with my son. I remember telling the officer that I probably shouldn't be driving. He agreed and asked me where I lived. He told me to be careful.

On the way back to the hospital I noticed people taking walks and smiling. In my frustration and grief, I couldn't help questioning their "normal" activities. Why didn't they realize my son was in the NICU with a terminal condition? I couldn't stop wondering, "Were they ever told their child was going to die? Have they ever lost a child?"

The results of Simon's hearing test revealed he passed in his left ear but required a referral for the right. I wondered if he was deaf in his right ear. His nurse, Olivia*, tried to calm me by saying "It's okay, a lot of people only hear out of one ear." Sandy, Simon's night nurse, was even more positive about Simon's hearing ability. Every time Grandma Lois snored, she said, Simon's big blue eyes darted around to discover the source of the noise. When Grandma stopped snoring, Simon would suck on his pacifier and close his eyes. Sandy said she had to stop herself from laughing so she didn't wake Grandma Lois. Maybe Simon could hear better than the test gave him credit for.

We wanted to take Simon home, and we continued to ask his medical team about that possibility. They said that babies don't typically go home while receiving infused medication. Prostaglandins, they added, are a short-term medication used before a patient undergoes surgery. They were also concerned about Simon's infection risk. His medical team advised us to consider stopping the prostaglandins so that nature could take its course. We resisted this advice because we believed their approach amounted to pulling the plug on our son. As Simon's parents, our responsibility was to guard and defend him. Simon's nurse *Beth asked us if we would like a meeting with the hospital's Ethics Committee. At this meeting we expressed our passionate desire to offer him the very best medical care available, and take him home if possible. Simon's medical team approved our decision to take Simon home on prostaglandins and stop his treatment at home.

Their best medical opinions about Simon's future left little hope. They thought that if we stopped the medicine, his PDA would close and Simon would pass shortly after. If we stopped treatment in the hospital and took him home, he would probably die within 24-48 hours. We still believed taking our little boy home was the best choice for him and his family. At least, at home, we could spend a few days with him. We were deeply disappointed to learn doctors didn't even plan on ordering more than a day or two of medicine for Simon. We expressed our disappointment forcefully to the Ethics Committee.

Scott was especially frustrated by the inability of Simon's physicians to share any concrete opinions about our son's best treatment options.

"Frankly, they never wanted to tell us squat," he said, still smarting from the lack of compassion he noted in some of Simon's doctors. *"I believe they saw Simon's condition as a hopeless case, and so they weren't interested in prioritizing his care. In one meeting when I had simply 'had it' with a constant litany of 'I don't knows' in regard to how Simon would respond to surgery or adapt to more hands-on care, I blew up."* Scott confronted them, stating angrily, *"You guys remind me of the weatherman, you don't want to go out on a limb on any decision!"*

It was hard for us to cope with the unknowns the medical team presented us. If these experts didn't know how Simon would respond to specific treatments, how could we feel confident making the decisions which confronted us daily?

Miraculous news intervened before we had to make the agonizing decision ourselves to bring our baby home for his last days on Earth. On October 14, Simon's echocardiogram revealed that the PDA was closed. We had prayed for it to stay open because doctors told us this was Simon's best chance to get the vital oxygen he needed in his blood. With most Trisomy 18 babies, the PDA will stay open on its own. We were relying on the prostaglandins infusion he received to keep it open.

When doctor Zandra came in with the results of the test, he said, "The PDA is closed." I cried and said, "No!" Dr. Zandra tried to comfort me by telling me, "This is good because the blood is still flowing through Simon's heart and he is getting the oxygen he needs. Someone else made this decision for you." I asked him, "Was it God?" Quietly, but firmly, this sensitive healer offered, "I believe so."

Prior to that amazing event, I learned one of his physicians planned to discontinue this medicine on his own. At that time, I confronted him. He insisted he would have checked with us first. How could I know that for sure? During that stressful period, caregivers often advised us to lower his dose or stop Simon's prostaglandins infusion. What if this had been Simon's only lifeline? Would the doctors have been willing to restart the medicine if the PDA did close? How could we be sure? Was Simon not a candidate for this life-supporting medication simply because he had Trisomy 18?

Right after getting the news from Dr. Zandra, Simon's medical team had another team meeting. They were amazed that Simon's PDA had closed while he was on prostaglandins. Dr. Zandra, a Hindu and spiritual person, put it this way months later:

"The closing of the heart vessel was truly amazing — extremely rare for the vessel to close without withdrawing medication," he explained. *"In my years 25-plus years of practice, I don't remember seeing it happen, and it has literally changed my clinical approach in treating babies with these kind of chromosomal conditions. It was not the medical team making the decision to withdraw medications — it was a much higher power, and I believe little Simon was consulted on that decision. He was always telling us what he wanted."*

We thanked God because cardiologists couldn't explain Simon's changing condition, as Dr. Zandra admitted. We knew God had His hand in this. Our prayers asked that Simon could soon go home and continue to live with us. Dr. Zandra had even said, "You may have him awhile." We would utilize Samuel and Sean's pediatrician, Dr. Ginnter*, as Simon's doctor when we went home. She agreed to follow up with echocardiograms as part of Simon's care.

Our first reaction to the echocardiogram was worry. But on second thought the issue that brought us great fear was now a tremendous blessing because the difficult decision to take him off the prostaglandins had been made for us. How? Apparently, the coarctation (thickening) of Simon's aorta was mild and therefore adequate blood flow could still get through the narrowing. Thank you, God! Simon was truly our little miracle man and no longer burdened with an IV line in his foot. Scott was equally thankful for the Lord's intervention, and he later told a group of men about his belief in the power of prayer in Simon's life during a retreat offered by our church:

"For Sheryl and myself, those drugs were his lifeline since it kept his PDA open and blood flow constant," Scott explained. *"We agonized over the decision to take him off the drug since we thought it might expedite his demise. His cardiologists told us that if the PDA closed he would most likely die. Almost every time we met with one of Simon's medical team, we had to emphasize that we would not make any decision that would expedite his death. When we finally got comfortable with*

removing the prostaglandins, a new echocardiogram was ordered. The results showed that the PDA was already closed, probably had been for some time, and Simon was still doing well. God does answer prayers!"

Simon constantly reminded us how to be strong, and he continued his fight to be with us as long as possible. We asked our friends, family and Caring Bridge prayer partners to ask the Lord that Simon suffer no more apnea episodes. Dr. Zandra had said, "You may have him a while." These were the best words we could ever hear. Still, we couldn't get too excited because Simon's doctors continued to say, "Simon will tell us his story." Despite their words of caution, it was still wonderful to think about the possibility of taking our precious son home.

Our most precious hope was that Simon would get well enough to go home with us. By October 17, we knew this plan was premature based on Simon's developing condition. The previous night Simon had four apnea episodes. He was struggling to get enough oxygen.

I spent many days facing the window. Simon liked the sun to shine in his room in the mornings. I loved to hold him, rock and pat his bottom. This was so comforting to him. As I looked out the window I imagined a patio and pictured myself holding Simon outside on those sunny days.

CHAPTER EIGHT

Promising signs

"Even the average pediatrician with a practice of 2,500 patients will only treat one trisomy child. Incidences may be relatively rare, but I always teach new physicians that children with chromosomal conditions haven't read the statistics. These families deserve an informed and thorough discussion of the challenges and options they face." — Dr. Stephen Braddock, director of medical genetics at Cardinal Glennon Children's Medical Center in St. Louis

After a difficult and emotionally exhausting weekend, Simon displayed some positive signs over the next few days. We believed an apnea monitor belt strapped around his chest may have triggered Simon's breathing struggles, and we asked that Simon be put back on the hospital monitor. We were testing the belt and monitor for possible home use when we achieved that goal, but the belt's placement around his chest seemed like a problem to us. Simon continued to grow and his apnea episodes subsided for a few days after double-digit incidents over the weekend.

Simon enjoyed his bath times in his little plastic tub. Boy, did he respond to that experience! Previously, his PICC line meant we could only wipe him down with a wet cloth. Finally, we could take our time pampering him with a normal bath. Our job was to do what made him happy and comfortable.

Other than a few heart rate drops, the next few days were great for Simon. However, in late October, he had an apnea episode, a frightening and heart-wrenching experience. We continued to live in the moment and prayed continuously for God to give us the maximum time with our precious son.

For a proud mother of a newborn, it's a frightening shock to have a hospice representative talk to you about your baby. We met with Wings, a pediatric hospice and palliative care agency that provides only one hour of nursing care a day in the home. We compared this level of care with the 24-hour nursing care completely covered by our insurance that Simon was receiving in the hospital.

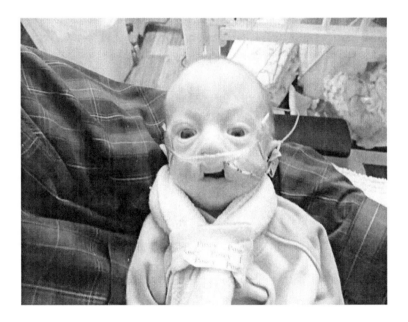

The Wings caregivers painted a beautiful picture. I wanted to pack up my little guy and go! Why couldn't I just pick him up and put him in my van and go home? After all, for nine months, while I was pregnant, Simon did live in our home. If

I took him home now, I could go for stroller walks with Simon, and he could finally adjust his beautiful eyes to the sunshine outside. I imagined taking him to the park next to our house and walking to school (just in back of our house) with Simon in the stroller.

Yes, Simon would still need oxygen. When we tried to reduce his oxygen flow, he didn't do well. Simon needed that little bit of O2 assistance. Another challenge was the thought of Simon having apnea episodes at home. What if we were having a stroller ride, and he had an apnea episode requiring the free flow or the bag and mask? After the Wings representatives left, I asked Simon's nurse about the bag and mask. She said we wouldn't have one. I asked, "What if he has apnea? She said, "That's a chance you take." How could I take a chance with his life? Some medical professionals would say that would be his time to go to heaven. Let Simon tell you his story, was their opinion.

We simply disagreed with this approach. Why wouldn't we intervene? Could we watch our baby struggle to breathe? We believe God has his book of life and only He would determine when Simon went to heaven. In the meantime, we wanted to offer the same level of care we would provide to any human being who needed it. If our approach failed, we were content not to advocate an overly aggressive response such as CPR that risked breaking Simon's fragile ribs. No one would convince us to simply ignore our son's suffering and stand by helplessly saying, "Oh, maybe this is Simon's time."

Did we even make the right decision about CPR? After all, his medical team led us in this direction. We had faith in our doctors, but was our faith justified? We were aware that some Trisomy 18 kids lived for months or years after being born with the syndrome.

Although Pam Healey's son Conor, who had Trisomy 18, died in infancy, her observations of long-term trisomy survivors has spanned 20 years of attending SOFT conferences. The Ph.D. researcher has studied 69 families with children who have trisomy conditions. The ages of the children were one to 21, with 19 at least age eight. This included 39 in the study with full Trisomy 18. Her experience with these families led her to a more optimistic outlook than is common in the field. Dr. Healey called movingly for a more family-oriented approach to critical medical decisions. In a recent article, she wrote:

"Day-to-day experience makes the parents the experts, the ones to educate any clinicians who will listen. They have anecdotes, journals, pictures and videos that tell, not of limited cognition but of development, meaningful interaction and joy. They have witnessed behavior that transcends the diagnosis. They have experienced love that transcends the disability.

"It is the people living with the long-term survivors who have the answers about the future, not the neonatologists or pediatric surgery teams who have never spent real time with older kids with what some call a fatal diagnosis."

When I insisted, the home care team found a self-inflating bag and mask we could use to assist Simon on stroller rides and car trips when we took him for checkups at his pediatrician's office. There would be no free-flow oxygen like he had available in the hospital. I thought about digging the hospital's more sophisticated equipment out of the trash. But I was warned that the hospital's equipment required proper training to use. I thought this was silly, since I was already using this same equipment in the hospital on Simon. In fact, I'd been trained on everything to do with his care, including feeding tubes, oxygen, monitors and the free flow and bag and mask. Besides, our nurse anesthetist friend Valerie lived just down the street.

When I allowed the social worker to go ahead and put Wings in place, Scott became upset. He said that the insurance company was not kicking us out of the hospital. After a phone call to our insurance caseworker, Scott learned that our insurance company actually preferred we stay in the hospital. The caseworker said that if Simon was still struggling with apnea, it was medically necessary and insurable for Simon to receive inpatient hospital care. We began to think our best option, at that point, was to stay in the hospital where little Simon had 24-hour medical attention.

"My only goal with Simon's care was that the doctors would treat his health issues with the same aggressiveness as they would treat a child who didn't have Trisomy 18," Scott explained. *"I didn't think they should put the burden on the parents to do the research about this rare disease with no information about the survivors who do exist. It too often felt like they were playing a shell game with our son's life — withholding information that might have convinced us to seek out more proactive treatment."*

I began to wonder about the wisdom of my desire to take Simon home. Was I even in my right frame of mind, making this decision without my husband's agreement? All decisions, especially Simon's care choices, were made together.

Going home would cost $1,000 a day for private-duty nursing. Although at the time I was willing to pay any price, I realize today we could never have afforded that level of care. Who could? Also, if Simon continued to endure constant apnea episodes, how would I ever sleep? I needed to function for my entire family! Even the nurses work 12-hour shifts and then sleep. I remember this conversation with one of Simon's doctors who said, "You don't get sleep with newborns anyway." I replied, "What if I'm so tired that I don't move quickly enough when his apnea alarm goes off?" He said, "Well then, that may be his time — let him pass comfortably."

Given the number of apnea episodes Simon had to overcome, we decided to stay in the hospital. There he could get 24-hour care from a highly trained medical staff. He simply couldn't get this care at home. I would be his primary care giver if we brought him home. I would feel so responsible if something happened to Simon while I was alone. What if Samuel and Sean had to watch him suffer and struggle for life in his crib while their mother panicked? What if we got Simon home and he only lived a few hours? What if Simon died in our home and our boys were afraid to go into his room after he passed? So many worries!

One of Simon's nurses, Lola, later endorsed our decision to keep Simon in the hospital, while adding her passionate hope for a more family-centered approach to high-risk infant support:

"Staff need to be more sensitive to parents and what they need," she said simply. *"So many things we think we control, God is controlling. I had three months working with this sweet baby that God gave us. I respected Scott and Sheryl — they chose to take the hard steps that were best for Simon. At the same time, there was a tough atmosphere among the nurses and physicians. We were not all on the same page. Someone needed to tell Sheryl that it was okay to keep Simon in the hospital — she was doing what was best for him and her family. She needed the support and structure of the hospital for her own well-being."*

A medical team can lead you down a path you don't want to follow. We continued to be proactive and challenge anything we were uncomfortable with. Not everyone shared our beliefs and faith, but we remained convinced our decisions were guided by God and Simon's best interests. We heard stories of some parents who chose not to feed their baby if he or she had Trisomy 18. This saddened me.

Still, the hospital was very accommodating. Simon's room became a true home for him and his family, with 24-hour care. Our son had some wonderful primary nurses. We continued to balance our two homes. The boys had a new kind of normal. Scott and I decided that, at that moment, this stable environment was best for our sweet Simon.

Halloween was coming soon. Our friend Jackie bought each of our boys at least three costumes. The boys were so excited because they love NASCAR and Samuel wore his Jeff Gordon costume with pride. Sean put on his Dale Earnhardt Jr. costume. Simon was Fred Flintstone but he drove a car, too. Pam, his nurse, made his costume. I guess she was falling in love with our little man. Simon wore a soft green necktie from physical therapy to help support his neck. His head wouldn't drop forward as much and slowly he built up neck-muscle strength. Pam put blue material over his green necktie and made him a darling orange and black costume. Who knew that Fred Flintstone's necktie was blue. Pam made sure of the color.

My friend Jackie Khalil later told me how comforting it was to observe nurses like Pam caring for little Simon. Jackie said:

"The most special memory I have of Simon occurred when I met him for the very first time. I recall Pam, one of Simon's nurses, talking to him very softly while she changed his diaper. He looked directly at her face and smiled with his amazing eyes. It is still a very vivid image in my mind the way he told the nurse, 'thank you for loving me,' with that one glance and those very captivating eyes."

Of course, Pam did not seem surprised by Simon's sweet way of communicating. She had the privilege of seeing Simon's extraordinary personality many times.

"My time at the hospital was an opportunity to see Simon's warm, calm and mature personality up close. But Simon's bravery and maturity are also captured in the many photos. You can see his trusting nature in the picture of Simon and protecting brother Samuel. All the photos of Simon snuggling with his family communicate the intimate way he expressed his love for them. I'm convinced by my memories of Simon and the photos I cherish today that Simon was wise far beyond his years. I believe he realized how fortunate he was to have a completely amazing and loving family here on earth and in heaven."

That weekend Scott would do what had worked in the past. If Simon was having apnea, Scott would say, "Come on Simon," and gently rub our son's forehead to make him blink. Scott would stop his nurses — especially if they weren't Simon's primary nurses — from immediately jumping to use the oxygen bag during an apnea episode. Scott knew that a calming touch and soothing voice might do the same thing as the bag — help Simon self-recover. Of course he would immediately ask for oxygen assistance if it became necessary. These nurses didn't know our Simon.

After a difficult Friday night and most of Saturday, Simon again showed his perseverance. He held his own. His brothers joined him for pictures in their Halloween costumes. Thankfully Simon was doing well enough that all of us took a break to join Samuel for his inspiring choral concert in Kirkwood.

Simon continued to gain weight, closing in on five pounds. His episodes were relatively minor that week compared to the previous weekend. Simon loved feeding time. He was always ready to fill his tummy a little before his scheduled time. He would offer a determined yelp to let his nurses know he was ready for his next meal. The doctor increased Simon's regular feeding amount, which seemed to make our little man happy. Last night Simon again mixed up his days and nights. He was ready to interact with Mommy and nurse Sandy.

We continued to meet with Simon's doctors. Every meeting I remember Scott saying, "We're not here to expedite his demise." There were times when the doctors and nurses thought we might be losing Simon. We remained committed to helping our little boy any way we could.

Through Simon, I've had the privilege of meeting physicians, scientists and nurses who don't automatically see trisomy-related conditions as "incompatible with life." One of those compassionate healers is Dr. Stephen Braddock, the director of Medical Genetics at Cardinal Glennon Children's Medical

Center in St. Louis and someone who I'm proud to call a friend. This experienced clinical geneticist recently explained to me his views on dealing with patients and families facing the challenge of trisomy-related disorders:

"When I counsel physicians and parents on the genetic implications as well as the treatment complications of children with severe chromosomal abnormalities, I'm careful not to sugarcoat the outlook," Dr. Braddock said. "The outcomes for these children are indeed grim, but the statistics that point to a 95 percent mortality rate are not an absolute death sentence. Things can happen — children do survive. Until I myself went to a SOFT (support organization for Trisomy 18, 13 and related disorders) conference, and had the honor of meeting these wonderful survivors and seeing the joy they brought to their families, I must admit I had never fully thought about that 5 percent who live meaningful lives.

"Think about the average physician who may never encounter one of these children," he continued. "The average neonatal team member will deal with some of these cases, but not in the numbers that build the experience and best practices to handle these situations with the greatest possible effectiveness and sensitivity. Even the average pediatrician with a practice of 2,500 patients will only treat one trisomy child if the numbers hold up. Incidences may be relatively rare, but I always teach new physicians that children with chromosomal conditions haven't read the statistics. These families deserve an informed and thorough discussion of the challenges and options they face. Children with trisomy-related disorders face profound disabilities, but every survivor I've seen interacted with their loved ones in a special way."

Dr. Braddock is right. When your child is the one fighting a chromosomal abnormality, he is 100 percent of your world. Experts like Dr. Braddock talk about living in the moment. We were doing exactly that. How could we not? We cherished every moment even as some caregivers kept saying Simon was going to pass soon and maybe he was telling us it was his time to go to heaven.

Once again, we focused on the moment. Our attitude was, "We have Simon now." He was such an unbelievable gift from God. Unfortunately, too often I remember certain nurses saying, "Well you know he is going to pass." Why steal our joy? We understood the ultimate outcome for Trisomy 18. We knew Simon could have heart failure. One nurse went on to say that I was in the denial stage and that Scott was in the anger stage.

When Heidi Drexler Photography came to do another family photo session, she offered her services free of charge again. Simon looked so adorable in his green and brown outfit with his rust colored hat. Simon was always a hat guy. The hospital auxiliary made so many cute hats. His nurses made sure he had one in every color. For our family pictures, Simon cooperated very well. When he made a peep, he got a drop of breast milk from his nurse.

Later, at a meeting across the hall from Simon's room, Simon's doctors told us the end was getting very near. Simon's saturation levels were falling. The alarm went off when Simon's saturation levels dropped. This was very scary because it meant oxygen wasn't circulating properly through his tiny body. Heart rate drops were also frightening because doctors told us Simon was likely to die from heart failure due to his damaged heart. Each alarm had a different sound, and every one made me jump. Many times the alarm went off when I was trying to sleep at night or when I was pumping breast milk. I felt constant palpitations and my own heart seemed to be ready to jump out of my chest. I reminded myself to take a deep breath and pray.

Another nurse, Sandy, would say Simon had an awful night. We knew this was true but the negativity in his room wasn't helpful. We feared Sandy was starting to listen to the "not compatible with life" crowd. On some days, Simon would really throw them off. These were the times when his nurses had to admit Simon was having a great day. Simon was going to call the shots, and we couldn't predict his will. We just loved and comforted him and stayed on top of his medical care.

When caregivers made thoughtless comments, we were hurt and frustrated. It seemed to us that if they weren't going to support us as parents, they had no business caring for our Simon. Didn't they understand it was an honor to take care of him and a privilege to meet him?

Simon's doctors often cited pulmonary hypertension as a major threat because of his complex heart defects. We were still confused at all the medical information flying continuously around us but grateful for Simon's nurses who took notes and explained Simon's changing condition in terms we could grasp.

We wanted to do all we could to keep our little man with us. Our goal was to never have him suffer but to question every medical decision and uncover choices we felt were being withheld from us. We wouldn't have chosen any treatment that might harm him, but we kept praying he would continue growing so he could receive life-saving heart surgery.

Simon's pattern then was frequent drops in his oxygen-saturation levels. That can be a sign of heart failure, pneumonia, or infection, or he could be aspirating. I asked the doctor, "How do we know what is causing the drops?" Dr. Essem* replied, "Well, what do you want to do? If there is an infection, are we going to treat him with an antibiotic? "I quickly replied, "Of course, I want him to have an antibiotic! Simon is our baby; he is a precious human being, and God will determine his lifespan." I then asked, "Isn't it typical to treat a Trisomy 18 baby with an antibiotic?" I wondered to myself, if the parent doesn't speak up, is the Trisomy 18 child denied an antibiotic? Does this life-and-death decision depend on the diverse opinions of different doctors?

Another neonatologist, Dr. Beller*, examined Simon. I was on the phone with Dr. Zandra at that moment, requesting an echocardiogram. Dr. Beller continued to examine Simon and decided to order an X-ray. I was encouraged that he ordered a test and didn't say, "Not for Simon." Dr. Zandra suggested we wait on the X-ray, and then do the echocardiogram. I believe Dr. Zandra always had hope for Simon. I always recalled his hopeful words, "You may have him awhile." At that point, anything positive went a long way with us.

Later, when I asked a nurse about the X-ray results, she replied, "The nurse practitioner said it was a crappy X-ray and that the doctor will read it in the morning." I asked her, "What the heck does a crappy X-ray mean? Is he okay? Is something wrong? She said, "The NP said it wasn't clear." I ended that conversation right then. I could do nothing but continue to worry. I needed an answer!

In the morning we found out that Simon was aspirating. The doctors ordered nothing by mouth until his respiratory issues cleared up. I was told that Simon wouldn't be able to receive his breast milk drops or enjoy any nursing or bottle-feeding. Simon loved breast milk. He found it so comforting and pleasurable. Of course, we needed to follow doctors' orders, and we wanted the best for our little man. His pacifier was the only comfort left he could take by mouth. We kept on snuggling him and giving him lots of love. This setback broke my heart because Simon was tolerating his feedings and gaining weight.

Echocardiograms were always frightening. We always dreaded the results. Simon's next echo showed a little improvement. Some of the medical staff took this as a positive and some felt it was not worth getting excited over. We took any improvement to heart. We even took the "no change" echocardiograms as a plus. We would never give up hope.

CHAPTER NINE

The journey home

"These parents have received the light of wisdom to realize that they are experiencing the kingdom of heaven within them when they take care of this child." — Bishop Robert J. Hermann

Our hope was built on the certainty that Earth is not our final destination. This is our temporary home. Although we were fighting with everything we had to help Simon live, we also gained strength from the sure knowledge that he would find his true home with Jesus in heaven. We believe that the right to life comes from the creator of life.

Unfortunately, too many people ignore the needs of trisomy children and others with severe disabilities. These children often can't speak for themselves. They are the most vulnerable citizens in our great country. Too many people are silent and won't speak up for these innocent children, unborn and born. Failing to protect the disabled is one of the biggest injustices in our world.

Simon's diagnosis of Trisomy 18 changed our lives dramatically. We lived in constant frustration that our doctors could share little information or reliable statistics about Trisomy 18. We kept hearing, "We just don't know." Each day we learned painfully that major medical interventions are routinely withheld from children like Simon. How would the statistics change if these children were treated aggressively? We wanted to give Simon every opportunity. After all, we would do the same thing for our other boys, Samuel and Sean.

Even though he continued to have a low heart rate and breathing interruptions (apnea), most days, physical stimulation combined with Simon's amazing tenacity helped bring him fully back. There were times when Simon needed free-flow oxygen (when a caregiver held an oxygen mask inches from his tiny mouth and lets it blow in his face) but his resilience demonstrated his desire to be with us every day. We never believed he was suffering or experiencing pain.

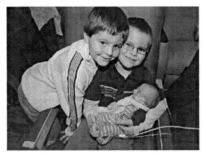

Although his doctors didn't expect him to survive the first week, Simon continued to live and exceed expectations. His spirit was so bright! He didn't even know he had Trisomy 18 with all its complicating medical conditions. He was so perfect and I'm so honored that God chose me to be his mother. Simon needed me and I needed him. Simon continued to teach me about the quality of life and how to live in the moment. He blanketed us in hope and joy every day.

We sought God's guidance in all of our decisions. This wasn't easy, but we tried to do what was best for Simon. Simon's number of days on Earth was up to God. We made sure repeatedly that the medical staff knew we weren't here to expedite his demise. I could see that Simon was changing people, especially some of his nurses. There was such a special place in their hearts for Simon. He felt their love and compassion and reacted to them with his captivating eyes and smiles. As one of his nurses said, "There is a reason his finger has a contracture (crooked finger). Simon hooks you."

Other friends of Simon were equally "hooked." Some of their comments capture that love and reflect a tiny sample of heavenly anticipation. Family friend LuAnn said: "I saw a small angel nested in his mother's arms when I first walked into the room. He had on his little green and yellow cap, with a smile that was truly blessed from up above. There he was at peace — an inner peace as if to say, "I know all the secrets of the universe, and they are so simple. Just look at me."

Valerie, a dear friend and certified registered nurse anesthetist, put it this way:

"Holding our precious Simon is a gift from God. He has a beautiful gentle spirit. It is so apparent that he has a deep connection to Sheryl, his mother. As I hold and rock him, he is restless and fussy. As soon as his mother takes him and places him close to her on her chest, so that he hears her heartbeat, he is totally calm and content. What a beautiful picture of motherly love. Simon is a blessing to all he encounters; I'm blessed to know him."

It was obvious to us that Simon loved life. He made the most of each day he was given. Each day was a gift and we were the recipients.

Another family friend, Cindy, saw the divine mystery in Simon's eyes. She said:

"The words that resounded in my mind when I first saw Simon, 'What are Simon's eyes saying to us — compassion and innocence.' I believe with all my heart that our Heavenly Father wanted to show us that we were privileged to meet, 'The Little Man.'"

Simon enjoyed life and looked forward to seeing his big brothers after school and those who love him. He recognized us, was alert and active and very aware of his surroundings. His big brothers were so in love with their baby brother and rushed through the hospital to 2264 Koala. Each day they took turns holding and playing with Simon.

As frequent worshipers at the Cathedral Basilica of St. Louis, Scott and I have had the privilege of meeting Bishop Robert J. Hermann, the Bishop Emeritus in Residence at the breathtakingly beautiful church. Bishop Hermann is a wonderful, soft-spoken man full of gentle wisdom and kind patience. He was brought up on a farm in southern Missouri as one of 15 children and his own nephew died as a child from complications due to severe brain damage at birth. The Bishop recently shared his own views on the role of special-needs children in God's eternal plan:

'These parents have received the light of wisdom to realize that they are experiencing the kingdom of heaven within them when they take care of this child. When we look at a special-needs child, Jesus is asking us directly, 'Do you see me?' These children draw out in their parents, strength and grace they didn't even know they possessed. They are a gift from God — to families, communities and the Body of Christ. Their ability to edify and inspire unconditional love can change our self-image from a culture of death to one that grants all God's children the dignity they deserve."

Yes, Bishop Hermann, my Simon inspired me to love more deeply than I ever knew I could. Oh how I loved kissing Simon's lips, his beautiful cleft lip. I also loved playing with his cute toes. I loved watching him breathe at naptime. I thought, "Our son is breathing — therefore he is living." If only I could still smell his precious skin and love on him all day long. What wonderful gifts he gave me. Simon was allowing us to keep making memories.

Simon's big blue eyes and big smiles always gave us hope. He was perfect in every way, and we continued to celebrate his achievements and milestones. The love and happiness that Simon embraced will always remind us all that Simon only knew love. His was a very special quality of life.

Simon was perfect with dark hair, 10 fingers and 10 toes, two ears and two big blue eyes. He had a beautiful little face and soft skin, long eyelashes and Daddy's eyebrows. He loved to kick his little legs and move his body around. He melted my heart every day, and I loved it when he clasped his fingers around mine and held on tight. I loved to hold his feet and see his toes move. There was so much to love about Simon.

Each day was a new day in Simon Land. We kept telling him how much we loved him and how proud we were of him. I think he was also proud to be part of our family. We loved to hear the music he sang to us with lovely noises accompanying the beautiful CDs that played in his room. He was always so peaceful and bright. It was reassuring that Simon noticed us and was always alert. He reacted and interacted and loved to have fun just studying our faces. He had an awesome personality, curious and wanting to know everything about his environment.

Father Joseph Jiang, then the associate pastor of the Cathedral Basilica in St. Louis, was born in China during a period when the Chinese government forced families to pay heavy fines or abort babies after reaching their quota of one. His life was spared when he moved in with his grandmother as a young boy. From his exposure to state-dictated values determining who lives and dies, Father Joseph was happy to express his passion for protecting the dignity of all life:

"The only perfection that exists in this world is God," the soft-spoken priest said slowly. "I can only grow when I begin to accept my own imperfection in the knowledge that every human being ever born, except for Christ, is infinitely imperfect compared to God. None us know the future, or when we are going to die. All of the plans we make, the material gains we accomplish, fail to define us or mark our value. What defines us is the love we express and receive at this moment. Love is the highest, eternal value that God recognizes. In that context, little Simon's contribution to the Kingdom of God was priceless."

To my family, withdrawing curative care when a baby has a diagnosis of trisomy is equivalent to a human rights crime. Isn't God the only one to determine the number of days we have here on Earth? I know that none of us are guaranteed a tomorrow. Why do some people think they have the right to life, but not all of God's children have the same right? We fought to make sure Simon was treated as an individual and given the same options as any other baby.

Simon was very much alive. Our son's desire to live was reinforced each day as he continued to prove himself by gaining weight and being alert. He smiled often and lifted his head. He wanted to see everyone in his presence. After all, 2264 Koala was his home. So we were confused why his doctors were so reluctant to offer specialized medical care. These are the attitudes that need to change for trisomy kids. Did some medical professionals not see him as a truly living person — especially after Simon was labeled with the most lethal level of Trisomy 18? Why do some caregivers use the awful term "incompatible with life?" Couldn't they see he was living?

It was very unsettling when medical professionals tried to make decisions without us. One doctor turned off Simon's saturation monitor and said, "We did this so you can enjoy him without the monitor making noises." I responded, "That's our decision to make." Even as we talked, Simon's saturation levels started to fall. Obviously, the monitor needed to stay on! I was in disbelief that Dr. Ritter responded to my decision by accusing me of being "mean." *Mean,* because I had the nerve to question him. *Mean,* so he responded unprofessionally. I was wrong for simply asking "why."

Other caregivers transcended these preconceptions about Simon's ultimate value. We were so grateful that these brave heroes consistently stepped up for our son. One doctor, Dr. Essem, kept leaving everything in our hands, asking, "What do you want to do?" When we gave him our answer, he would respond, "Okay then — that is what we'll do." It was deeply comforting to interact with a doctor who acknowledged our wishes as parents. It was a pleasure to meet a physician who practiced hope, rather than gloom. We were so robbed of joy during my pregnancy. Why couldn't we be joyful and cherish the hope that Simon would continue to beat the odds?

While we believed, for the moment, Simon was best cared for in the hospital, we did take steps to welcome our son home in the near future. Scott set up Simon's crib on the lower level of our home in Webster Groves. We needed to make sure that his oxygen source would be convenient and accessible. I also wanted Simon on the main floor so I could monitor him constantly. We continued our training with the home health company. Simon even passed a car-seat challenge, a study conducted by a physical therapist that ensured we could carry him in our car safely.

We continued to prepare for his life ahead. We needed his doctors to support his health first, and prepare for his death last, not the other way around.

Many did care deeply about Simon's positive progress. But sometimes we were confused as a gentle voice advised us, "Maybe Simon is ready to go to heaven now. It may be his time." Were his own caregivers in a hurry for him to die? We continued to ask many questions and challenged Simon's medical team. At times we struggled with their medical advice but had faith that God would continue to guide our decisions and Simon's ultimate fate.

As I sat in his room kangarooing Simon, feeling his heartbeat and embracing the warmth of his body, I wondered how the Trisomy 18 diagnosis affected his doctors. What really was their motivation? I believed that some had pure concerns for Simon's life but could muster little hope for our little boy. Were they signing Simon's death warrant before his time? It nauseated me to believe this. It wasn't fair for my precious son to be treated any differently than a full-term baby or even a Down syndrome child. After all, Trisomy 18 is second in occurrence to Trisomy 21 (Down). Unfortunately, not many people — even medical professionals apparently — know much about Trisomy 18. Simon's doctor kept telling us that he didn't know about his future. He explained that each child is unique with different medical complications.

After educating ourselves, we understood that it's not Trisomy 18 that kills but the resulting anomalies. How is it okay that only doctors are qualified to determine who is and is not compatible with life? When my dad had cancer, he underwent treatment until there was nothing more doctors could do. He was 57 when he passed. Simon was a baby who was also terminal. If someone, even a baby, is terminally ill with cancer, do they write him off and withhold medical treatment? Simon was a human being, a child of God and our precious son!

Simon's mission was to touch as many lives as possible. We hoped our family's love might overcome the negative predictions that rang continually in our ears. Simon and his medical needs were never a burden, and our family wanted our little man. Our Simon was very charming and so happy. He loved to hug, be bathed, play, kangaroo and just enjoy family time.

The positive energy of friends like Stacy always helped us to keep up the fight for Simon. She recalled a moving visit:

"Today I have the privilege of seeing Simon for the second time. With me is my video camera, to capture some special Simon moments. I walk in and see my dear friend Sheryl looking lovingly at Simon in his crib, moving his oxygen tubing to a more comfortable position. I'm truly amazed as to how this little guy, who I know is very sick, looks so wonderful! When I first visited Simon, I fully expected to see a frail-looking baby. Boy, how I was wrong! Today is the same. Simon has the brightest eyes staring back at us, tracking our every move. I hadn't expected him to be so alert and observant. It makes me smile! He's looking so intently at both of us as we rub his little toes and hands and as Sheryl recounts the day's activities with Simon. And then it happens — the hiccups! Both of us start laughing; they sure are loud for a little one! It's moments like this that make you stop and realize that even in such a solemn place like the NICU, there is a time for laughter to go along with the tears."

I found the emotional support of Simon's nurses and the spiritual outreach of the hospital chaplain incredibly uplifting. These visitors to Simon's room had no intention of being negative. They continued to treat Simon and inform us softly and respectfully while honoring our wishes.

Many days I felt the neonatologists were partnering with us as Simon's parents. We just wanted our wishes honored and not to be looked at like we were crazy for wanting our son to live with Trisomy 18. Simon's best interest was our only goal.

The neonatologists and NICU nurses were very good at encouraging bonding between baby Simon and his parents. After all, babies with short life expectancies most need love, care and dignity. Our neonatologists believed that noninvasive support and comfort care were appropriate. We tried hard to align our goals with his medical team to do what was best for our precious man.

I knew Trisomy 18 children who lived past one year existed. I loved to imagine Simon as a toddler. One night, I put Simon on the fold-down couch with me. So sweet — he had no idea what I was doing with him, especially when I laid down next to him to sleep. His nurse watched him on the monitor while we slept. When I asked nurse Catherine to get approval for this, she didn't think I was crazy. She agreed it was a lovely idea, a great memory to build. I didn't sleep but my baby slumbered soundly, and I watched his peaceful sleep with true happiness in my heart.

Simon continued to display his toughness. We were surprised when Dr. Ritter mentioned the possibility of a swallow test to check for reflux. I was excited about this news, so I shared it with Patricia*, one of Simon's nurses. Patricia explained that Dr. Ritter's plan could lead to speech therapists coming in to observe his bottle feedings.

Patricia's reaction was, "Really?" I asked if she was surprised by this news. Her only reaction was, "No comment." I then said, "You're surprised Dr. Ritter would order this test because Simon has Trisomy 18." Again, she replied, "No comment; I'm not saying anything." I know deep in her heart Patricia was happy that Dr. Ritter was ordering this test for Simon. Was Simon melting the experienced physician's heart? I asked myself, "Would some Trisomy 18 babies not be offered this study?"

Simon was already on Mylicon and Mylanta. His nurse Catherine was the first person to mention Mylanta for Simon's indigestion. I requested it, and the doctor agreed. The truth is, if you want something for your child, you may just have to ask for it. The medicine sure seemed to help Simon, and he loved the taste. I think he thought it was a treat when he tasted it.

Oh, how we anticipated Simon's two-month birthday on November 7. We planned to celebrate with all Simon's caregivers, big brothers and Grandma Lois. It was extra special because Auntie Judy, Scott's aunt, was coming in from Kansas City to meet Simon. Just about every day Auntie Judy wrote a beautiful heartfelt post on Simon's Caring Bridge site. She loved Simon before she even met him, and I know Simon loved her back.

On that day, Auntie Judy fell even more deeply in love with Simon. She spent the night in his hospital room with Grandma Lois and slept with one eye open to watch him all night. Her beautiful display of faith, hope and love was placed on his shelf in the form of a beautiful silver decoration. She also presented Simon a stuffed elephant in a Kansas State University warm-up suit. She said Simon was strong and mighty like an elephant.

Auntie Judy later wrote this special tribute to the little boy who changed her life:

"This is the blessing I cherish as I reflect on Simon Dominic Crosier. I think of the influence his valued presence and his loving soul made on

ever so many who embraced him and shared in his journey. The only space between Simon, his family and the dedicated medical family was clearly filled with hope. They loved him, held him and celebrated together each precious moment of life.

To hold him was to feel instant love. His gentle nature peered back at me through those blue eyes as tears filled mine. It was his two- month birthday, a joyous day of celebration and smiles. I was blessed to share this remarkable milestone with him and sing "Happy Birthday" to our dear little man.

My few days with Simon were quickly passing. It was then we shared one last snuggle "alone time" as my having to say goodbye was just a few hours away. As I held him, I noticed his left fingers had become somewhat more relaxed. With that I then placed my pinky within his sweet, tiny little hand and sang 'bye oh bye oh baby'...'your mommy is a lady'...'your daddy is a gentleman' and ...'Simon, you'll always be their baby.' God so blessed me to have had that moment of specialness.

Always with love and special memories,
Auntie J"

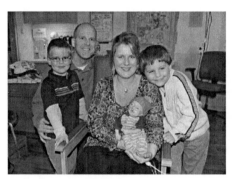

We celebrated Simon's two-month birthday all day long. We decorated his room with "Happy Birthday" signs and balloons bearing his name. We had fun taking photos of Simon in his birthday hat. His favorite photo op was with nurse Lola, one of his primary daytime caregivers since he arrived in the NICU. He also requested that we bring treats for all his wonderful caregivers in the NICU who enjoyed cookies and brownies courtesy of Simon.

Simon's weekend was mostly good with a few minor episodes. We continued to pray for comfort and strength for our awesome little guy. We were also excited that Simon surpassed the five-pound mark on the scale. On toward six pounds we go. He had also grown two inches in length since birth and was now 19 inches long. We hoped these growth trends could continue. We believe Simon's continued victory over his many physical challenges was a direct testimony to the many wonderful and powerful prayers he received.

Our little champion had great days and some rough ones. I still remember the night when *Lucy, his nurse, was stimulating Simon because he was having an episode. She had reached for the bag and it didn't look right to me. Fortunately, Simon self-corrected and started to breathe again. I mentioned to Lucy that the bag didn't seem to work properly. She said she would check it out.

The next morning, we told day nurse *Ellen about the situation. She agreed it was unacceptable to have faulty medical equipment and made a note to change the bag every couple of weeks. When she ultimately replaced the bag, I thought I noticed a hole in the old bag. This was a scary oversight since even a tiny hole could mean life or death for little Simon.

Ellen was always encouraging and supportive. I remember saying to her, "We just wanted a third child, and we prayed and prayed." She responded, "You have your third child. Simon is here!" It was so comforting to hear this.

The second week in November, Simon had another echocardiogram. We felt blessed that the results came back positive, reflecting a reprieve against the impending dangers his doctors were anticipating. Simon did wonderfully for several days, and we had a brief period of enjoying our Simon as a comfortable and content baby.

Simon continued to thrive, as he grew bigger by the day. He was 5 pounds, 4.3 ounces, or in metric terms, 2392 grams. Apparently his continuous feeding regime agreed with our little man.

We knew Simon's heart defects were complicated. His Trisomy 18 led to these cardiac medical complications. But after he received his two-month Vaccinations (diphtheria, pertussis, tetanus) he developed high fevers. Simon's baseline oxygen levels were never the same after these injections.

After Simon's two-month immunizations on November 14, his fever spiked to 102 degrees. His oxygen intake was also increased to one liter. By the next day, he was back down to .4 liters of oxygen and he seemed to be recovering nicely. Two days later Simon received the balance of his two-month immunizations, and his fever returned to almost 99. We insisted that his nurses give him Tylenol if needed. His oxygen needs again increased to .7 liters, and free-flow oxygen was administered.

The next day we placed an urgent request for prayers for Simon! His previous few days had been stressful for Simon and our family. The immunizations took a lot out of our tough little guy. The doctors had grave concerns about his pulmonary hypertension.

I firmly believe Simon's immunizations took a toll on him. I understood the reasons given for immunizing Simon. Samuel and Sean attended grade school where the daily chance of bringing home germs presented a real challenge to Simon's vulnerable defenses. Whooping cough was going around their school at that time.

Simon's next echocardiogram showed his heart had deteriorated. His oxygen deficit went up significantly and he was very pale. We thought we were going to lose him. The next day was a very precious gift. Simon's oxygen requirements lessened, and his color improved. He was attentive and interacted eagerly. He was still the sweetest little man ever, and we believed the prayers of his many family, friends and Caring Bridge fans were pulling him through.

Simon had already shared special holidays and holy days with his family. I arrived at the hospital for his delivery on Labor Day. We celebrated Sean's birthday, his two-monthly birthdays and Halloween. The next holiday to anticipate was Thanksgiving the following day. Our family was so thankful for our Simon.

Simon's night nurse Lucy even told him that tomorrow was turkey day.

"Simon, turkeys say, 'gobble, gobble,'" she told him excitedly. Simon looked at her and seemed to enjoy her imitation of a turkey immensely. When Lucy showed Simon the felt turkey with his name on it hanging by his crib, he got the full visual as well. When I thanked Lucy for taking such good care of Simon, she said, "It's an absolute honor and privilege to care for precious Simon."

As we celebrated Thanksgiving with our little boy, we expressed a heartfelt thanks to all who traveled this difficult journey with us. We said thank you to Jesus for blessing us with Simon. We thanked all the prayer warriors across the country that never even met Simon. Their support gave Simon amazing strength to fight every day. And our family gathered daily strength from these petitions as well. Thank you family and friends for the kindness and caring that kept us positive. The support we received in the form of gift certificates, greeting cards, meal pick-ups and big brother drop-offs meant everything! A simple thanks only touches the surface of our family's gratitude.

The week of December 2 wasn't filled with the positives we continually prayed for. Simon's oxygen needs increased while his heart-rate drops also became more alarming. Worst of all, his peacefulness and comfort were frequently interrupted.

One night Scott was awoken at 4:30 a.m. by a nurse practitioner. Simon was awake, fussy and clearly irritated. The nurse practitioner complained that Simon's nurses were unable to quiet him. "Do you want to give him morphine?" she asked. Scott knew instinctively that giving a powerful narcotic to a tiny infant with severe heart problems was a bad idea. We stood our ground and adamantly refused her recommendation.

Instead, Scott gently took our son in his strong arms and rested Simon on his chest. Our son calmed down immediately.

More than two years later, my friend Debbie Bruns, Ph.D, principal investigator for the largest study of trisomy-related syndrome survivors in the world, shared this bit of research with me:

"Anecdotally, parents with infants with Trisomy 18 and 13 have reported that morphine reduces or suppresses breathing. As such, morphine should be contraindicated for infants with cardiac and respiratory issues, which comprise the majority of those with Trisomy18."

On Dec. 2, Simon was fussy and upset. I tried holding him in many positions, wondering if reflux or breathing problems were causing him to be uncomfortable. His saturation levels were consistently dropping and I felt extremely helpless. Again, Melanie asked if I would consider giving Simon morphine. I couldn't believe it and I was quickly getting angry! "No morphine," I said. Instead we were offered a sedative, lorezepam, which slows brain activity and encourages relaxation. We were assured that this medicine would not have an impact on his damaged heart. During the last 24 hours of Simon's life, he was given this sedative twice to comfort him. I still question my decision to allow Simon to receive this medicine. At the time, we prayed passionately for Simon to have peace and for our family to enjoy God's grace.

CHAPTER 10

In the arms of Jesus

"We moved Simon to her, and this time she knew the end was near. It's all right for him to let go. I told the doctor, 'it's time.'" — Olivia, Simon's nurse

Our precious Simon went to rest in the arms of Jesus on December 3, 2010. When he died at 10:45 a.m., his transition to heaven was so surreal. I remember holding him and telling him, "It's okay Simon. If you want, you can go to Jesus." Then I yelled "Olivia!" for Simon's nurse, who was standing with Simon's doctor right outside his door. I yelled because I saw his oxygen saturation levels drop very low. The nurse called Scott. Time was now very short. Would Simon wait for Daddy to get there? Scott was approaching his office downtown when Olivia reached him. He immediately turned around and headed back to the hospital. Maybe our little warrior would wait for Daddy. Dr. Pang said Simon's heart rate had dropped to 40-60 beats-per-minute.

Thankfully, Scott arrived and held Simon peacefully in his arms. We could sense our baby slipping away. How much longer would we be able to love on our little Simon's beautiful body? Did Simon want both of his parents there with him? Scott eventually felt the warmth of Simon's body dissipate and escape as he embraced him.

The night before, Scott had spent the evening with Simon. I remember asking him if he could stay because I was so tired and didn't think I could make it another night. We believe that Simon, being his considerate and compassionate self, allowed Mommy a good night's rest at home with his big brothers. He was glad to have Daddy there by his side. Dr. Pang frequently said, "Simon was always so peaceful and thoughtful." Even in death, as our little man passed from this world to the next, he reached out to those he loved. Through the love and compassion that Simon was born to convey, he set the benchmark for God's presence in this world.

My memories of this moment are clouded by grief and helplessness. Olivia, Simon's devoted nurse, later shared her own objective observations of the dreamlike scene at the moment of Simon's death in the Koala pod, the only home he had ever known.

"Sheryl came flying in the room," Olivia recalled. "We moved Simon to her, and this time she knew the end was near. It's all right for him to let go. I told the doctor, 'it's time,' when I left the room for a brief moment. Then I heard 'Olivia, Olivia!' When I raced back into Simon's room, I heard Sheryl telling her precious baby it was okay to go to Jesus. Simon was on her chest. When I turned the monitor off for the last time, I knew Simon had only a few minutes to live. I wanted those moments to be in the arms of his loving parents.

Simon's friend and devoted comforter continued, *"I had promised to take Simon downstairs when the time came. Dr. Pang listened for the heartbeat, and Simon was with God. I believe in my own heart that I actually felt his immortal soul leave his body and I'm thankful I was there for that."*

Olivia, Simon's defender until the end, escorted our little man to the holding area where his tiny body would await transport to the funeral home:

"I emailed Simon's team of nurses thanking them for their help," Olivia recalls. "As my colleagues came into the room to say goodbye, I stayed at my post thinking it was my fate to be here at this moment — I was meant to be Simon's nurse and it was meant to end this way. I knew I was going to be by his side when he finally passed. Visitors — mostly Simon's caregivers and nurses —in those hours after his death had to go

through me. I served as the gatekeeper as Sheryl and Scott took the time they needed to say goodbye."

Olivia protected Simon — and us.

"Some hospital staff asked why we were waiting to transport Simon's body to the holding area," she said. "I reassured Scott and Sheryl that they should take as much time as they needed. When my shift ended at 7 p.m., I stayed, finally telling the security escort that I would take Simon downstairs as if he was my own child. I carried his lifeless body to the ground floor on my shoulder swaddled and warm. When asked, I responded forcefully that the family desired no autopsy be performed."

Olivia understood perfectly when Scott and I explained why the boys were not coming up to Simon's room, even though some hospital staff questioned our decision. Our reasons were sound. Samuel suffered from anxiety and depression. "Mom I'm mad at you. You didn't let us say goodbye," he said. "Mom and Dad did what was right," Sean replied. "Mom knows best." Still, Samuel wanted to know why we didn't get him out of school. We didn't want the boys to remember Simon like that.

After breathing his last breath in his Daddy's arms, Simon's monitor was finally turned off and his feeding and oxygen tubes removed. Simon rested in the arms of Mommy and Daddy until 8:15 p.m. that evening when nurse Olivia carried him to the hospital's lower level. Scott and I knew that by the end of that evening, our son would be alone in the funeral home. As I look back, I wonder how I could have allowed brave Simon to be alone. Yet I know Simon was never really alone.

As the reality set in of Simon's passing, we struggled with how to tell our eight and six year old sons. We asked ourselves, "How do we deliver the horrible news?" We even consulted with our pastor. As a mom of two young boys, how cautious did I need to be for their protection? Their little hearts had become gigantic for Simon. The passing of their little brother forever changed their lives. As a family, although we had known the grief and frustration of losing six babies to miscarriage and enduring Simon's brave battle for life, we never gave up hope. We picked up our other two sons, Samuel and Sean at our friends' house after we left the hospital. They lived only two miles from St. Paul's Hospital that had been Simon's home for nearly three months. Samuel and Sean visited their baby brother Simon every day after school. However, this day was different. They went to be with friends, and Simon had gone on to heaven.

Our dear friend Stacy was watching the boys at her house before we arrived to bring them to the park. She described the scene:

"Today is December 3, and Samuel and Sean are at our home playing with our kids while Scott and Sheryl spend some special time with Simon. He's had a tough week, and the doctors fear this will be his last day. I hear the doorbell ring; it's Scott and Sheryl at the door with tears in their eyes. Precious Simon has lost his hard-fought battle. I give Sheryl a big hug and try in vain to keep from crying myself. None of us wanted Samuel and Sean to know what had happened just yet.

"Scott and Sheryl so want to protect them from the reality that the little brother they love so much is gone. Sheryl walks numbly upstairs with me as we look through my children's dress clothes, trying to find suitable outfits for her boys to wear to little Simon's funeral. She has small bursts of emotions that come out, but overall she's holding things together. How, I don't know. Scott is downstairs with my husband, Lou, trying not to let on to the boys what has happened to their baby brother. The boys are asking how Simon is doing, but the truth will have to wait a bit longer, until they have a private place to talk, just their family. There is so much love in this family, and I know that they're all going to be okay because of that love and their strong faith in God."

As soon as the boys got into our van, they immediately said, "Let's go see Simon." At that point we drove to nearby park. Samuel knew something was wrong and asked if Simon died. We told him "yes," and he went running as fast as he could, screaming and crying onto the playground. Since it was dark out, there was no one around, and we knew this was probably a suitable place to break the devastating news. Our boys needed the open space. We stood there, holding and wrapping our arms around our sons.

That night when we got home, our evening was filled with non-stop crying and holding one another. As a family of four, we committed that evening to always hold on tight to our family. One thing Simon taught us is that it wasn't about Scott's and my needs. We made it about Simon and Samuel and Sean. They coped with Mommy at the hospital, but they both reassured me, "Mommy, you would be with me, too, if I was in the Koala Pod." My boys agreed that Simon should never be alone. So many family memories; were they enough?

That Saturday morning, Scott and Grandma Lois went to the funeral home to make final preparations for Simon's funeral. We decided to put Simon's picture on the memory card. So many people had prayed for Simon, but never met him. His card said:

In Loving Memory of Simon Dominic Crosier
September 7, 2010-December 3, 2010

"We believe God saw Simon was getting tired. A cure was not to be. So the Lord put his gentle arms around our son and whispered, 'Come to me.' With breaking hearts we watched him fade away. Although we loved him dearly, we couldn't convince him to stay. A golden heart stopped beating, hard-working hands to rest. God broke our hearts to prove to us: He only takes the best."

The next two days were a blur. Relatives came in town and helped prepare for Simon's day of honor. Auntie Judy and Grandma Lois did a fabulous job getting photographs together of Simon for display at the visitation. Since we decided on a closed casket, we wanted plenty of photos and Simon's favorite things on display. Among the items were his beautiful quilt, favorite *blankies,* stuffed animals and his mobile. This is the world Simon knew. Part of his big spirit will always fill his room at St. Paul's NICU, Koala 2264.

On Monday, December 6, 2010, about 4 p.m., the phone rang. It was Dr. Fiore's office from Cardinal Glennon Children's Medical Center. I made this appointment with the cardiac pediatric surgeon while Simon was still alive. At that time we still believed heart surgery could save his life. Unfortunately, we had forgotten to cancel the appointment. It was painful to tell the doctor's assistant that Simon could not be there.

The next day, we arrived an hour before the visitation. Finally, Samuel and Sean had the time to say their goodbyes. Seeing Simon in his little 19-inch casket was heartbreaking. He looked beautiful in his blue outfit that said, "I am awesome, like Daddy!" His little cleft lip was even more noticeable to the boys — probably because the ever-present oxygen-carrying tube was no longer dividing his nose and mouth. We cried and held one another up as a family. We comforted one another by reminiscing about how awesome Simon was. Sean had always called him "Super Simon," even before he was born. He was truly a fighter. Father Bob Evans, our parish priest, also prayed with us. Father Bob assured us that God didn't make Simon sick. "Simon is in heaven," Father Bob reminded us. "He is no longer afflicted with Trisomy 18 or heart problems."

When the funeral director told us it was 11:30, we knew the last hour of our time with Simon's physical body had passed. We walked back into the parlor and the visitation line began. It seemed endless. We were surprised to see so many people. The experience was a bit of a blur with lots of hugs and condolences. In the background, the recording star Selah's CD played — the same one Lola, Simon's nurse, gave us right after he was born. My favorite song is "Carry You." The lyric says, "I will carry you while your heart beats here. Then

Jesus carries you and I will praise the One who's chosen me to carry you."

As we entered the chapel for Simon's service, the finality of the event became more real. Our sweet, precious Simon was not physically here with us anymore. I noticed Simon's picture with Father Bob holding him on the altar. Another parish priest, Father Mark Dolan, delivered a homily about God's creation. He called Simon our Saint. Samuel and Sean brought up the gifts for Mass. Our two little men seemed lost in a blur of introspection and sadness.

Next, was Deacon Bill's beautiful memorial to Simon. I don't think there was a dry eye in the chapel. Below are some of his moving words as he spoke on Simon's behalf.

"Dear God I know you, I have seen you, I have been held by you, touched by you, my family introduced me to you. They loved me as you love me now; you and they are one. What can I say to ever express what has happened to me in my short stay on earth.

- *Thank you, thank you, and thank you for knitting me in my mother Sheryl's womb. (Psalm 139)*
- *And God, how can I find a way from here to thank mom and dad for giving me life even when they knew I would not be perfect and might not be with them long.*
- *Wow, what a gift those 88 and a half days were.*
- *You know God I was loved perfectly just as I was by mom and dad, by my brothers and by so many others.*
- *God, do you know what it is to be held and cuddled — and just loved for who you are and it did not make a difference if I messed in my diaper or made a fuss or cried real loud I was just loved.*
- *And now here I am with you God, oh how can I ever say thank you to all who loved me into being and gave me the gift of who I am.*

"God's response: You know, Simon, I think you already said thank you by just being Simon for that is all I ever hope for from anyone who is born. If each person is loved into who I created them to be then they will be happy and I will be, too. You see, Simon, your life is not about you; you are about exposing love, and you are about exposing Me, God. The incarnation goes on every day, wherever love is experienced, Jesus is present and I am revealed. Thank you, Simon, for loving them all, as I love you. And Simon, one more thing, the love you experienced will never end. You will see them all again, and we all shall be together forever."

Another close family friend, Lisa Mills, helped express Simon's role as a messenger of love from heaven in this tribute to Simon she wrote after visiting him in the hospital.

"Simon — so small, yet you impacted so many lives. Such a brief time here on earth, yet what a ministry. From the time we knew Sheryl was expecting Simon, he taught us the importance of trusting God. His presence in St. Paul's impacted all of those who knew him as he radiated God's love. The brief visit I had with Simon was such a joy and one I will never forget. What an example of God knowing the whole picture; Simon's impact then, and his family's ongoing impact and ministry to others who suffer. As hard as it was on those left on earth, Simon is complete, whole, and will enjoy God's presence and perfection for eternity. Thank You, Lord, for bringing Sheryl and Simon into my life.

Thanks for making love Godvisible."

Godvisible. It's a word like *Godincidence* that describes the unconditional love we had and still have for Simon. He will always remain with us, reflecting God's love in our memories through his beautiful wise eyes. Surrounded by their cousins, Samuel and Sean kissed Simon's coffin. Samuel looked up smiling and said, "Simon's in paradise."

We felt a tremendous void after leaving the funeral home and driving to the cemetery for a private family ceremony. We thought having the visitation on the same day as the funeral would be easier on the boys.

When we arrived at Resurrection Cemetery, the chapel was prepared for his celebration of life. Yellow roses with ribbons designated "Beloved Son, Brother and Grandson" were laid upon his casket. Simon Dominic Crosier is buried only a few miles from our home. After my father, David Florek, passed November 30, 2002, Scott and I bought our own plots next to Dad. Simon is buried at the head of my plot. As his mother, I needed to know our connection on Earth and in heaven would last forever. Is any mother ever prepared to bury her child?

Simon lives in our hearts, and our arms will always ache to hold him. In the song "Cry With Hope" by Steven Curtis Chapman, which Scott's sister Staci sang at the funeral, the words say, "We can cry with hope, say goodbye with hope because we know our goodbye is not the end. We can grieve with hope, we believe with hope there's a place where we'll see your face again. "

It's that same hope and our faith in Jesus that keeps us going. The grief we experienced is present every day. After Simon's death, it was very difficult to have a conversation with anyone. Not only did I struggle to comprehend people. I stuttered. I had never stuttered before in my life, so I know this was grief-related. It was very embarrassing because I couldn't control it. I prayed that my stuttering would stop. Grief has many emotional symptoms — and a lot of physical ones.

Samuel and Sean's Bible study teacher and our dear friend, Dona, said it best in a card. "Grief will be yours for a lifetime until you are all reunited again with Simon and all your babies. Don't let anyone rush you through it. Crying is good for the soul."

At the visitation, I remember Simon's nurse, *Lilly, saying she felt the Holy Spirit in Simon's hospital room. Others had also told us that his room was sacred. That's why we fought against negativity in Simon's room. We all sensed it was a gateway to the divine — sacred ground. Mary wasn't Simon's only nurse who sensed a spiritual aura surrounding and protecting our precious man.

Catherine said all the nurses were "Simonized." They had all been permanently changed by their interactions with this special boy. "To this day, I think of it as Simon's room," Catherine said recently. "His innocence in the face of great physical distress was a kind of miracle. He never did anything wrong, and we all know he never would in his short stay here with us."

Mary later told me a story that sent a chill down my spine and reassured me that Simon knew Jesus personally even during his short stay on Earth. This deeply faith-filled woman described it this way:

"On the third day of looking after Simon, my husband drove me home after a long shift at the hospital. When my husband was born, doctors immediately said there was no hope for his survival, but he grew up into a loving, healthy and Godly man. As we drove in silence on mostly deserted streets early in the morning, we came to a church on the corner of Ballas and Manchester. On the steps of that empty church, as clearly as I have ever seen any member of my own family, I saw our Lord Jesus Christ. His arms were open in a welcoming gesture and the words soundlessly entered my heart — 'Simon is in my arms.' At that moment I had no doubts. Little Simon was in the care of our Savior."

We read this and will read this every Christmas as a family:

My First Christmas in Heaven

I see the countless Christmas trees around the world below
With tiny lights, like Heaven's stars, reflecting on the snow
The sight is so spectacular, please wipe away the tear
For I am spending Christmas with Jesus Christ this year.
I hear the many Christmas songs that people hold so dear

But the sounds of music can't compare with the Christmas
Choir up here. I have no words to tell you, the joy their voices
Bring. For it is beyond description, to hear the angels sing.
I know how much you miss me; I see the pain inside your heart
But I am not so far away, We really aren't apart.
So be happy for me, dear ones, you know I hold you dear.
And be glad I'm spending Christmas with Jesus Christ this year.
I sent you each a special gift, from my heavenly home above.
I sent you each a memory of my undying love.
After all, love is a gift more precious than pure gold.
It was always most important in the stories Jesus told.
Please love and keep each other, as my Father said to do.
For I can't count the blessing or love he has for each of you.
So have a Merry Christmas and wipe away that tear
Remember, I'm spending Christmas with Jesus Christ this year

Wanda Bencke following the death of her daughter Lysandra Kay

We posted on Simon's Caring Bridge site, "Merry Christmas Simon. Hope you had fun celebrating Jesus' Birthday today. We love you, we miss you and we think of you all the time. Love, Mommy, Daddy, Samuel and Sean."

Christmas night we were praying and talking about Simon celebrating Jesus' birthday in heaven. We imagined Simon at the table with Jesus having cake. Then Sean said, "I bet Simon is dressed up like *Buzz Lightyear*." We all laughed.

A few weeks later, on Valentine's Day, Simon revealed himself in the form of an ice sculpture shaped like a heart. That morning Simon's big brothers, Samuel and Sean, noticed the heart on our deck and said, "Look Mommy, Simon sent us a heart for Valentine's Day." What a great way to start the day. However, the joy didn't last for Samuel. At the class Valentine's party, a mother brought in her baby who was Simon's age. Grief strikes us all differently as Samuel experienced at the party. Another mom who had attended the funeral was also at the party. This memory was much too fresh for Samuel. He told me later that the mom stood behind him holding her baby on her chest saying, on behalf of her baby, "Hi Samuel, Hi Samuel." As the baby lightly touched him, my grieving son struggled with his emotions. "She must have thought I didn't care if I had another brother," Samuel explained to me. "I want my baby brother, Simon." Samuel added he was eating his cupcake with his fists tightly closed because he wanted to run away. He said all the girls were telling the mom, "Oh, your baby is so cute." Samuel said, "I excused myself to the bathroom because I just wanted to hide."

Unfortunately that day's substitute teacher didn't know about Samuel's situation, so there was no opportunity for him to express his sadness and confusion. Samuel just kept his head down while participating in arts and crafts. Samuel wanted to enjoy the party, but this day was very difficult for him. Wouldn't it be difficult for any eight-year-old who lost his baby brother?

Let's face it — most people who haven't gone through the loss of a child may not be very comforting. They may say something like, "But your brother is in heaven" or "There are babies everywhere," because they don't understand. Our family was still mourning the loss of Simon.

After prayer and talking with grief counselors and social workers, I requested that the school notify me if babies would be present in the boys' classroom. I felt compelled to protect my sons and give them the emotional space they needed. It seemed wise to remove them from the classroom for a time whenever a baby would be present. The teachers were very sympathetic. The Clark School principal, Mr. Bill Schiller, was very compassionate and willing to work with us. Mrs. Gibson, Samuel's teacher, regretted that she wasn't there to protect him. The next day, Samuel said to his teacher, "Bummer you missed the Valentine's Party." This was also his way of saying, "I trust you and you would have understood my feelings."

Sean's teacher, Mrs. Boone, later told me that protecting the boys was a priority at their school:

"My primary thought was to alleviate stress and pain," she explained. "For Scott and Sheryl, the best I could do was to support Sean and make things as consistent as possible for him. I gave him endless opportunities to talk about Simon. We displayed Simon's picture and footprint in the classroom. We would have daily updates and as a class we celebrated Simon's good days and experiences that helped Sean think of his brother as being like any other baby."

Bill Schiller is no stranger to grief and the loss of a child:

"Having lost my daughter, Anne, at the age of ten to a four-year battle with a nasty brain tumor is not something I generally think of as a plus in the life column," he confided in me. "I do see it as an experience I have had that allows me to be very supportive in situations like Samuel's and Sean's. I had shared my experience with Sheryl who shared it with dad. They encouraged Samuel to talk to me. My main message was: It's sad. It doesn't seem fair. These are hard things to figure out how to handle. I narrowed it down to two choices. One choice would be to let this event stop you from growing and becoming a better person. The other would be to decide you were going to be the best person you could be. What would Simon want? Would he want you to have a good life or a bad one? (That answer always seems clear to kids and adults). So then do what Simon would want. It doesn't mean forget Simon or you can never be sad. It does mean you can do those things and then step forward to having a life where you still grow while remembering the good there was about Simon. As I said, I try to take my very difficult experience and help support others through theirs. It doesn't make sense to waste my experience and hide it away when it can support others."

Mr. Schiller was instrumental in Clark School's decision to erect a playground bench and tetherball set in Simon's honor. Mary Claire, a Clark student, has also received a grant to dedicate a tree in front of the school with a stone bearing Simon's name. In the fall of 2011, at the commemoration service unveiling the memorial and honoring Simon, Bill Schiller talked to me about the role of community in handling grief:

"The death of a younger person is something that sticks with people," he said. "Maybe it's because we hope and believe it will never happen to our community and more specifically to us. When it does it seems to waken the good in people. We are more supportive, more understanding, more willing to lend a hand. I believe that the families and students in Samuel and Sean's grade levels (and many others) will remember the hurt they saw in their friends. Having the bench, which is a useful item on a very busy playground, is a very fitting remembrance for the Crosier family. The bench honors Simon and his family. At the same time, it's now an interwoven piece of playground community life. What has happened to them is something they won't forget. The bench is one of many reminders of that for them. It is also a reminder that life is active and always moving and growing. The bench is part of the active community life of Clark, and so then is Simon and the Crosier family experience."

Not only do we suffer as bereaved parents, but we also carry our surviving children's pain. You try to do the best you can to protect your children. We ensured that appropriate counseling was available. The world goes on and people don't understand. Perhaps they don't want to take the time to understand our situation. We don't know what's in their hearts, but we do know what compassion is, what suffering is. The emotional support we received decreased after Simon died. People saw us out and about and thought, "Oh, they're doing well." The truth is you must keep going for your surviving children. But what you really want is to sit in the corner and cry all day.

It's hard enough seeing babies Simon's age. In time I'm sure the hurt and pain will soften. But at that time, I needed to go through the grief — not over or around it. I was physically sick when I saw a baby or even a pregnant woman because I was wounded. Even with the pain, I would never undo the pregnancies with the babies we lost to miscarriages or Simon's birth with Trisomy 18. God gave all these babies life in and out of my womb. All seven of these dear souls are now in heaven. In the arms of Jesus, Simon no longer suffers with Trisomy 18, and his heart is brand new. Our hearts continued to be broken. God didn't make him sick. God knew the number of days Simon had here on Earth even before our little man went back to heaven.

I was very uneasy about the future — months that Simon would never experience here on earth. People said, "Oh, you were so blessed to have him as long as you did." Within his first few days of life, we were confronted with his imminent death and advised to plan his funeral. How many people, especially the ones who have never experienced a loss of a child, would really cherish each and every day and then say, "It's okay. At least I had my baby for a short time."

When I was pregnant with Simon and terrified about some of his troubling ultrasound readings, a neighbor actually came into our garage and said, "It would be better if **IT** died."

We didn't get many Caring Bridge posts from people anymore. Once someone passes away, I guess people typically stop visiting his website. We chose to update journal posts about our life after Simon passed, and some of those thoughts or incidents are shared with you in this book. We want you to be aware of the miraculous signs that Simon is communicating to his friends and family.

For example, Samuel and Sean now call 1-800-Jesus. This all started one day when Samuel made this comment: "If Jesus was here walking the earth, I would call him on his cell phone and ask him to go to Koala 2264 and fix my brother Simon's heart." We told the boys they could call Jesus in heaven, too. So Samuel and Sean dialed up Jesus and asked for Simon Crosier every day. Usually this happened as we tried to get out the door for school. You wouldn't believe the fun Simon is having in heaven. Not only is he a NASCAR driver, he also parties in his room with his friends and his sister Sophia. He enjoys bowling, baseball and baby spa time with as many massages as he wants! This is the imaginative world Simon's big brothers live in. Scott and I cherish the chance to join them there.

But the world keeps going. It doesn't stop for people like us. We don't move at the pace of others. We take it slowly. This was our Simon grief time. We wanted to talk about him in our mourning. Compassion has to be taught. One has to experience trials to grow. I bear the battle scars, and it's always a blessing to meet others who share our insights. I've learned to look beyond the moment and ask the big question. What am I being taught here on earth, and how can I assist others?

I visit Simon most days, and as a family we visit him every weekend at the cemetery. We have pictures of our special baby and put out fresh flowers by his grave for each season. It hurts so deeply to know that the youngest member of our family went before us.

For his grave, we chose a stone with prayer hands. We'll never forget Simon's big brothers noticing his prayer hands when he was in his crib back at the hospital. He'll always be our beloved son and Samuel and Sean's baby brother.

A neighbor asked me how I was doing, and I told her it was very difficult. I said some days were better than others but there was still so much hurt. She said, "It'll get easier and you'll heal. Simon is in heaven and doesn't have to suffer anymore." I appreciated her good intentions but thought, Simon didn't suffer the way people believed he did. His doctors would have agreed. He was always peaceful and pushing ahead to the next challenge.

My neighbor had never lost a child, and she merely reflected the way of the world, which is, "Let's move along." I said to her, "The boys are hurting. Simon was their baby brother, and they're grieving in their own way." She said, "Yes, but they will get over it." I thought, "**it,**" get over "it?" This was our Simon, a beautiful human being.

Others make well-intentioned statements like, "Oh, I didn't say anything to you because I didn't know he lived that long. I thought he died at birth or shortly after." Comments like this make me wonder: "Do people think less of a baby's value if they're stillborn or die shortly after birth? People also often say, "He was so small and fragile." Well-meaning comments can cut like a two-edged sword. Because he was fragile and small, does that it make it okay that he is gone? We miss our Simon, special needs and all.

My husband, a man conditioned by his Midwestern Lutheran upbringing to hold his emotions deep inside, penned this beautiful poem at Simon's passing. He shared his father's love and pride for Simon with the whole world.

Simon's Prayer

Jesus blessed us with a beautiful baby boy
Despite many ailments, he brought so much joy
He was strong and tough and fought till the end
Simon is his name; he is our son, our brother, our friend
Our blessed Simon so sweet, so innocent, so pure
Your short life had great purpose we know for sure
It was hard to let go because we loved you so much
But thanks to prayer, we have a way to stay in touch
The magnificent kingdom of heaven is now your new home
One can only imagine the beautiful places you have to roam
The arms of Jesus must feel amazing and fit you like a glove
But your greatest gift on earth was your unconditional love
Till we see each other again, you will burn bright in our hearts
In eternal life you must be happy and healthy with all perfect parts
But be sure to be listening as we pray for you to intercede

You're our little saint; every word from you will be special indeed
May you send us daily reminders of Christ's presence in our life
Reminding us of his love and directing us away from strife
In our hearts and souls your memory will forever burn bright
And with a forever heavy heart I bid you a restful good night

CHAPTER 11

Life after Simon, you don't get over HIM

When you're told that your child is "incompatible with life," your world shatters. But when you find the truth and know there are other divine messengers out there only hoping to connect, the Lord shares his blanket of comfort and hope.

It's really nice to be supported by compassionate people who've heard the insensitive comments or tired clichés themselves. Support groups for the loss of a child validate your emotions. So do the few moms I've met who've lost their own babies to Trisomy 18.

I went to an infertility group last night at the St. Louis Archdiocese and met some wonderful people. It was the Archdiocese's annual infertility Mass, which was followed by a wonderful reception. These brave would-be parents may not share our experiences exactly, but they're hurting, too. They want a child and have been unsuccessful. Each month becomes a deeper-felt loss for them as they continue to grow older. There are even couples who receive grants from the Archdiocese for adoption. I'm deeply touched by the options these selfless couples are willing to pursue with faith and hope. Catholics typically come from large families, but how about some empathy for these suffering souls who can't have children?

I know one of my directives from God is to have compassion for these brothers and sisters in Christ and to help them walk their journey. Isn't this what all of us are called to do in the Body of Christ?

I met a compassionate obstetrician at the reception. I briefly explained our situation to Dr. Dixon. He said, "So you're probably asking me, what do I do with the last eight to ten years of fertility." I told him I never thought about it that way. All I see is that I'm now 42 years old. I assured the doctor that our family would never have changed anything. We were so blessed to have Simon. It's true, I added, that it just hurts so much now that he's gone. We continued talking about the value of all human life. He said, "You and your husband never said 'No' to God."

As we parted I thought of my other babies who never came to term. We cherish each of them by name and had special intention Masses said for each of them. They're also human beings with innate dignity and value.

We planned a golf tournament in memory of Simon for August 20, 2011, at Spring Creek Golf Course in Seneca, Kansas, Scott's hometown. Our goal was to raise money for Trisomy 18 and keep Simon's name alive through the contributions of family and friends. Scott's cousin Amy lost her baby to Trisomy 18 when she was only four-months pregnant. We're proud to invite all those who have lost their babies because of Trisomy 18. We also welcome those special survivors and their families who are still living with this life-affirming challenge.

As my heart continues to yearn for Simon, God has offered me a wonderful gift. It's a pure love for trisomy children and their families. I recently found out there was a baby born with Trisomy 18 at a local St. Louis-area hospital. I dearly wanted to hold this baby! One of Simon's nurses passed on the news that another Trisomy 18 survivor was born at a local hospital in November. Speaking on behalf of these precious babies, allow me to say, "Yes, we Trisomy 18 messengers from God may be rare, but we're perfect in the Lord's sight. We're special visitors from heaven."

For those trisomy survivors who are still here on earth, praise God. They're a gift to the world and to their families. They're going to visit us on Earth a little longer. But we'll all meet again in heaven because we've been promised that reunion through the resurrection of Jesus Christ.

We all need to embrace the strength of love that comes from an unexpected crisis. Every crisis is a family crisis because we're all part of God's family, the Body of Christ. Our country needs families who value life, because we're all connected. Our connection is woven through faith, family and hope. Unfortunately, I see these God-given virtues being torn apart right and left. We must stand together and cherish each and every human life, no matter how short.

My circle of friends, the core of my community, all try to understand. But their lives go on. After the first few months of life without Simon, I wanted to be stuck where I was. I was grieving. When I was alone, I could be still and know that God is God. Our feelings are important to God because he created us and wants us to be whole.

We all want to be loved, understood, defended and protected. Scripture says we are to weep with those who are weeping. We are to carry our brothers' and sisters' burdens when they can't. When people don't have compassion, when they're so focused on their own lives, how can they reach out?

Living in the moment with Simon taught me a lot. It doesn't matter what people do. Who you have in your inner circle means everything. If we ask, the Lord will provide us with wisdom and discernment. Yes, it would be a great world if everyone could be a rock for one another, like Simon Peter and our own little Simon. But that's not the world we live in. Alienation is the force that too often moves our Earthly existence. We must protect our immediate family and battle, on our knees, if necessary.

I see things I couldn't see before. I see people for who they are and who they're not. Toxic people are like saltshakers on an open wound of the vulnerable. Self-preservation and protection became our defense mechanism. We learned that we couldn't engage with even close family members who didn't support us, and at times, brought negativity into our lives.

On our path, He places *Godincidences* everywhere. I don't push my feelings away anymore. I'm aware of my emotions. I know what I'm experiencing and, yes, it's often painful. It still hurts to see pregnant women and babies because my grief is very deep. But I take the time for self-care and I embrace my pain. The Lord has also allowed me to embrace pregnant moms with the prenatal diagnosis of Trisomy 18. I've been privileged to hug their Trisomy 18 babies. I can relate to these families. I have been there, too. Being a chapter chair with SOFT is a ministry in itself.

I know what is happening and I trust Jesus. I hope to show more compassion to others. It is that understanding that I can wrap my heart and mind around. We hold close our treasured memories and continue to make memories in Simon's honor.

My family lives in the moment with the Lord, as we lived each second with Simon every day God blessed us with his presence. If I don't stop to feel and recall these precious moments, if I sweep my feelings under the rug for the sake of others, how can I have compassion and wisdom? I want to stay in the moment now and observe my Simon's nudges and signs from heaven.

Fear is a feeling I now observe with compassion. When you're told that your child is "incompatible with life," your world shatters. But when you find the truth and know there are other divine messengers out there hoping only to connect, the Lord shares his blanket of comfort and hope. He asks us to practice kindness and compassion with ourselves, and others. I still feel the sadness and loss, but I can pay it forward by being an advocate for all trisomy children.

Life is both rewarding and challenging, especially for the vulnerable. Because of Simon, I'm more aware of those blessings God puts in my path and my relationship with the Lord is so much deeper. Before Simon, I may have not noticed others because I was living in my own little world. I pray for those who are hurting and want to include them in my life. I can no longer ignore their sorrow. I know what it's like to be ignored. I've wiped my tears away as uncomfortable, and unengaged friends and family simply walked on by. I want to be the Good Samaritan who stops to help those in need.

People don't want to talk about the dead, especially babies. I believe these angels have gone to prepare our way. If we focus on eternal life we know we all count! Someday I may be ready to move on as people often urge me to do. But when I do, Simon is coming along with me. My prayer is really for those who meet people like me, people who are grieving, and don't say anything. Acknowledgement and concern can help us carry our heavy load. Compassion goes such a long way. The Lord calls us to exercise mercy. I believe compassion and love really can be learned.

Simon helped people learn about suffering by connecting to others, some of whom he never even met. He was a precious angel with a wise soul. He taught us unconditional love and compassion. So if I weep, allow me to weep. I'm aching for my son. Deep in my heart, I rejoice because my hope is in the Lord. I will hold Simon again!

Simon's pictures are everywhere in our home. Sometimes, in the stillness of a long sleepless night or a quiet afternoon, I can feel him on my chest. It helps to listen to Simon's music, hold his clothes and look at his pictures and keepsakes. Writing this book, I can experience intense feelings because of the continued connection I have with my son. I reminisce about Simon looking at me with his big bright blue eyes. Simon's eyes were portals to pure divine love. Meantime, we'll carry Simon's memory forward with our annual Simon Dominic Crosier Memorial Golf Tournament. We'll also watch our "Simon Tree" grow and grow. This tree is on the 11th hole in the backyard of Scott's parent's home on a golf course in Kansas.

We all have jobs while we're here on Earth, as we will in heaven. In the Bible, Paul teaches Timothy about God-given gifts. I pray that my family is being formed into something that is more Christ-like. We've become advocates for children with Trisomy 18. I want to share a couple of organizations that support these families. One great investigative arm for learning more about trisomy survivors and their families is the Tracking Rare Incidence Syndromes (TRIS) project. The chief investigator of that organization has been blessed with an amazing gift — true empathy for kids with Trisomy 18 and their parents.

This organization is run by Debbie Bruns. She is a researcher interested in children with rare trisomy conditions. She later explained to me the path that took her to her current work tracking children and adults with Trisomy 18:

"After teaching young children with significant developmental delays and medical conditions for five years, my doctoral research took me into the neonatal intensive care unit," she explained. "I never forgot the three girls in my classroom with Trisomy 18. Doctors might not believe there are many survivors with Trisomy 18, but there are. In the early 2000s, I virtually met many families with living children in Australia, Canada and the United States. (You'll meet some of those survivors and families in the Afterward of this book.) In January 2011, I received a call from a brave Missouri woman named Sheryl Crosier."

Through my contact with Debbie, I was eager to share our story with other families with a child with Trisomy 18. After three months in the hospital, Simon's records consisted of 4100 pages. Reproducing would have cost 50 cents per page; but I then called Dr. Pang, and he sent us a nine-page summary. We wondered why we would have to pay so much for our deceased baby son's complete medical records.

One mother I met had a beautiful daughter with Trisomy 18 named Molly. Molly lived for two months in the ICU at St. Paul's. Molly's mom told me she sensed people wanted healing for Molly so *they* could be less uncomfortable.

When people haven't lost a child, they can never fully understand. Instead of saying, "I understand," it helps more if they try to be a good listener. I wanted people to ask about Simon and let me tell them how much we missed him. I wanted to tell them all about Simon in detail, and really hear me! Don't try to change the subject. We appreciate and cherish our friends who genuinely care and want to listen.

Others may say to be thankful for your other two healthy boys as though they want to redirect the conversation away from Simon. I now respond, "I can be thankful for Samuel and Sean and still miss my Simon."

So many times I feel loneliness, and my arms ache to hold Simon. I yearn for that day to hold all of our babies again. For now, we have memories of being pregnant with our girls and also carrying Simon in my womb. We had 88 1/2 days of joy with Simon Dominic Crosier here on Earth. In this lifetime, we'll continue to cry with hope. Because as the song says, "We know our goodbye is not the end." Sean expresses his own vision of his little brother's current status beautifully, saying, "Jesus is telling Bible stories to Simon in heaven."

Since Simon passed, I've had many vivid dreams about Simon. The first was on a Saturday in January, and I was at home wondering why I wasn't at the hospital. Then it occurred to me that Simon had gone on to heaven. But when I went to the hospital, I found him in his crib in 2264 Koala. I rushed into his room and picked him up. In my dream, Simon no longer was burdened by oxygen or feeding tubes. I kept kissing him and telling him how much I loved him. I carried him around the NICU and told everyone that Simon still lived. He hadn't passed away! What was everyone thinking?

My second dream was in late February 2011. This was also lovely and peaceful! Behind our house is the school our boys attend. In my dream, between our house and the school, was a pond or a pool. I couldn't quite make it out. Simon was in it, floating and smiling at me. I picked him up and smiled at him, saying, "Simon, we have to pick up your brothers from school." I was already 10 minutes late. So I took off his oxygen and carried him along the pathway, which had many trees, to the school.

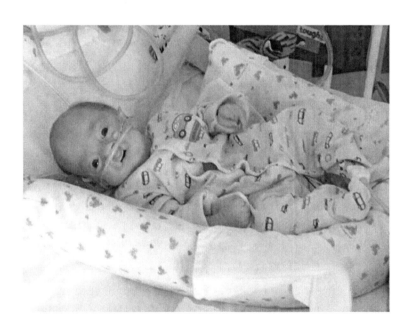

I kept saying, "Mama loves you." Then we'd look into each other's eyes and he'd respond, saying his own name — "Simon." Simon could talk! We repeated this several times and his eyes sparkled, so big, blue and beautiful. Then Simon said, "Are we at Daddy's work?" I said, "No, this building is your brothers' school. It looks so big to you, but it isn't downtown where Daddy's office is." Then Samuel and Sean came out of the school building and we rushed home.

Simon dreams have never been restricted to his mother. One night brother Samuel had the most beautiful dream about Simon. In his dream, he heard someone knocking on our front door. It was Simon in a tuxedo. Yes, dressed for success! Samuel said that Simon also had a translator with him. It must have been Simon's guardian angel, since they were here on earth. Samuel said that Simon came in, and we kept kissing him. Wouldn't this have been the most awesome dream come true! For our family it would have been paradise.

Simon's nurse Olivia says she has met our Simon in her dreams as well.

"I was at work, and it was close to the time for him to be with God," she says of her dream. *"After he passed, I saw him in heaven with his siblings — joyous and grateful. It wasn't a coincidence that I was assigned to him. In those three months, lives were changed and souls were touched."*

In September 2011, I had another dream in which my little Simon told me he was doing just fine in heaven. Simon looked so sweet just staring at us. He had no oxygen, and he was talking. Daddy had him in a pumpkin seat and was rocking him. Then Simon said, "I want you to hold me, so I took him out and held him so close. Mrs. Davidson, Samuel and Sean's school nurse, was also Simon's nurse in my dream. She reassured us that everything looked good with Simon, and added she saw no problem after studying Scott's X chromosome inversion. She said she'd never seen anything like these DNA strands before. We also went to Kansas with

Simon, and he was having a ball at Grandma Lois' house. He was talking, and everyone was snuggling with our little man. Simon kept staring at a wall where many animal prints were displayed. It was the same kind of print that Simon had in Koala 2264 on the curtain in his room.

In special dreams like these, God's little messenger brings us hope and comfort. Simon's moments on this earth are saved and protected in our hearts. Our unconditional love for Simon will live for an eternity. Nothing can take it away! But until we meet up with Simon in heaven, our hearts will ache for him. The promises of God's word are so comforting.

In Matthew's gospel, Jesus says, "Blessed are those that mourn, for they shall be comforted." The hope we have in Christ Jesus provides us with a peace beyond all comprehension. It's the peace of knowing with absolute certainty that our Father's arms are holding Simon close. Together, they send a special grace to the broken-hearted.

That grace also came to my family in the comforting words of dear friends. In a card from Catherine, one of Simon's nurses, she said, *"He was a special angel and will always be with you. He has a perfect body now. No Trisomy 18 or cleft lip. You'll hold him again someday. My brief encounter with Simon left me a changed person. We'll all miss him. Thank you for the opportunity to care for such a special baby."*

Lola, his primary nurse, wrote:

"I truly believe we came together by 'divine appointment.' Simon's life has affected so many other lives. It was truly a blessing to care for him. For now, our time with him has been put on hold. Although he cannot come back to us, we will one day go to him. I look forward to seeing him again — and I'll know it's him when I see those big, beautiful eyes!"

Our friend Margaret sent a very special note. Having lost a daughter herself, she wrote:

"Your life is separated distinctly by the event, 'Before Simon and after Simon.' What comfort you may find with God, our Father, who knows exactly how it feels to lose a child. Simon is resting comfortably in the arms of his Savoir, Jesus. I do believe that God shed the first tear for Simon and take heart that He knows how painful your tears are. He entrusted Simon to your care in and out of the womb. And, as his parents and brothers, you witnessed to all —God's immeasurable love. Simon surely felt this abundant love and care, and he will never know a day without the love of Jesus. Unfortunately, I know of this pain, and I will not let you walk it alone."

What a disciple of Christ Margaret is! What a comfort to us! She is a friend who has freely chosen to walk this journey after Simon with us! It's people like her who make the world a brighter place, when the grief process can be so dark.

Simon taught us about purity and innocence, but his brothers are carrying on the lesson for him. Recently, Sean said, "I would like to take Simon's place." I explained to him God's book of life. Only the Lord knows the number of our days. I know both Samuel and Sean would give anything to be with Simon — as would his parents.

Simon is our bright shining star. After his parent/teacher conference, Sean came bounding up our condo stairs and pointed to a single shining star in the sky. Samuel immediately went over to look and said, "Look, it's Simon!" We believe that Simon is watching over his brothers and all they do at Clark Elementary. Simon also says: "Thank you Clark for all you do for my big brothers." We took this special opportunity to take a picture of Simon's star as it shone right behind our boys' wonderful school.

Where there is hope, there is life. We would say this a lot when my Dad was going through cancer treatments in 2002. The term used for Trisomy 18, "incompatible with life" is so very harsh and is meaningless when you have faith in our Lord. My Dad died at age 57. Simon had 88 1/2 days. It doesn't matter how long or short a life is. God calls us to cherish each one of his creations. Just as Auntie Judy's Caring Bridge post said, "Dear Simon, 'How blessed we are for a lifetime of love we have for you.'"

March is Trisomy Awareness Month, and March 18 is dedicated to Trisomy 18. We'll keep these children and their families in our prayers. In addition to Trisomy 18, other rare chromosomal conditions challenge our ability to treat our brothers and sisters as we would be treated. Some of these children have lived much longer than Simon. There is hope for these angels. For Simon and others who lived only a short time on this earth, there is the sure knowledge that we will see them again. They're waiting for us in heaven.

CHAPTER 12

Grant us peace — give us courage

It's very clear to me that Simon's treatment would have been different if his medical caregivers knew he had Trisomy 18 before his birth. We would never make a decision to withdraw care. If Simon had been diagnosed with Trisomy 18 while still in my womb, we would have still insisted on the fullest, most appropriate efforts to bring him to term and care for him after birth.

Happy six-month birthday Simon! It was March 7, 2011. We hope you enjoyed our visit and when your big brothers let their blue-star balloons go up and up and up. Samuel and Sean hope you received them because they wanted you to have something to play with.

The expressive therapists from Wings, the bereavement group for kids, visited with Samuel and Sean a week later. They asked the boys to draw a picture of what they would like to see Simon doing in heaven. Samuel drew a tropical resort and a tiki hut. Simon was driving around the resort in his racecar. The picture shows Simon going down the water slide into the hot tub. Then our physically unhindered son dives off the board into the water. When he gets hungry, he goes to the tiki hut to have breast milk. Sweet-tooth Sean chimed in at this point — "and cookies!"

In his picture, Sean drew a heavenly golden racetrack. Except Sean's heaven is re-named "Simon's Cool Gold City." Sean said God was driving Dale Earnhardt, Jr.'s racecar. Simon was in God's pit crew. Simon had sunglasses on because the gold was so bright. Also, Sunday was Samuel's Kirkwood Children's Chorale concert. His favorite song was *Amani Utupe*. Appreciating the world around us means also appreciating the diversity of people that live here. "Amani Utupe na ustawi" translates as "Grant us peace, give us courage." Such beautiful voices! Samuel knows that Simon enjoyed their singing.

The other day I was trying to imagine my life before I was even pregnant with Simon. I know I was grieving the loss of our babies to miscarriages. Every time I seemed to lift my chin up that old wound re-opened. I guess it never really healed. As my friend Silvia said, "You are being pulled out of the operating room and never went to the recovery room. People just want you to move on and — in the well-meaning but inadequate word — "heal."

Many times, I feel like I'm still pregnant with Simon. I can feel him move. I feel my husband's touch, the warm hands of Samuel and Sean on my belly praying for our Simon. If I could have known Simon would only have three short months on Earth, I'd ask God to keep me pregnant another nine months before delivering my special son.

During the boys' school spring break in March, our family traveled to what is now a magical landmark for us. You see, this location carries the same name as our little guy, St. Simon's Island, Georgia. We spent the first half of the week in St. Augustine, Florida, enjoying many of the sites and history of the oldest city in the U.S. Everywhere we walked we had our Simon with us — not just in spirit — in a laminated 8x10 photo that we included in our family photos of the trip. We stood in victory lane at Daytona International Speedway, toured the World Golf Hall of Fame, and learned a lot about Timicuan Indians while touring the Fountain of Youth grounds in St. Augustine.

After a wonderful time in Florida, we drove north up Interstate 95 to stay at the King and Prince Resort on St. Simon's. It didn't escape our attention that we had always referred to our little boy in royal terms while he was with us. St. Simon's is an absolutely beautiful place that combines native Georgian trees with beautiful palms more commonly seen in the tropics. We enjoyed the beach, bike rides, pool time, the Georgia Sea Turtle Hospital, and an absolutely amazing sunset that Simon surely sent our way.

Our view of life has changed forever. We'll never be the same after Simon entered this world. We found a little slice of heaven when we went to St. Simon's Island. Our son's beautiful name was everywhere, St. Simon's Elementary School, St. Simon's Eye Care, St. Simon's Sweets, and more. I think I was running on emotion and adrenaline. I felt peace and a comfort that I had not felt since his passing. Simon was truly with us! The signs said "Little St. Simon's Island." How fitting! Little St. Simon's Island for our "Little Man."

During our travels there, I read John MacArthur's book, *Safe in the Arms of God*. He states:

"God knew precisely how long your child would live and for what purpose your child would live. Your child's destiny was and is in His hands. God superintends and guards every life He allows to exist. He places every life into context of His eternal plan and purpose."

I appreciate this author stating, "My heart grieves with any parent who loses a child, and that's what motivated me to search Scriptures on this subject so I could reach out and offer biblically founded words of comfort and encouragement."

Many times, MacArthur says in this wonderful book, our babies have "instant heaven" when they pass. I couldn't agree more! We continue to make memories together and keep Simon always close to us. Simon's love for us, and the signs he continues to share are sources of joy. They're as real as the beautiful Georgia ocean sunset Simon sent our way. We look forward to the beauty we'll all share on the day of our resurrection.

We marked Simon's seven-month birthday in April! "Dear Simon, your big brothers said you have been eating yummy cake all day long. Samuel believes there is an unlimited supply of cake and breast milk in heaven. Samuel and Sean sent you a birthday balloon from each of them. Outside we watched the wax candles we made with our special notes inside burn. Your big brothers enjoyed sending you their love notes. Please Simon, give them a sign you received their balloons and notes."

We were thrilled that our children's devotional scripture reading for April 7 started off with Simon's name! In Luke's gospel Jesus says, "Simon, Simon! Satan has asked to sift you disciples like wheat!"

Sean said recently, "I think Simon wants us in heaven." I tried to offer my living son this consolation: With death comes separation. But once the Earth is restored, there will be no more death. We'll meet Simon in heaven, and then when Christ returns, heaven and the New Earth will be one. Sean even says, "It will be like the garden of Eden, before Adam and Eve ate the apple and disobeyed God." Sean is right on!

Death had separated us. One day we'll be re-united in heaven and then we'll make up our lost time with Simon on the New Earth. We'll watch our babies that were taken from us grow up. How awesome is our God! Oh, how we miss him and how I still feel him. Our friend Lisa Mills was visiting with me at our home. I love to share Simon's pictures and his room with those who had such a love for him. I remember saying to Lisa that day, "Why didn't God take me with Simon? Wouldn't that have been wonderful if I would have been able to go with Simon?" Lisa just looked at me and said, "It was not your time yet."

At home, Simon's room is the place where we feel closest to our little man. All of his items from Koala 2264 have been placed in his special room. It touches my heart to see Samuel and Sean in this sacred place for quiet reflection time. Sean likes to go through Simon's clothes and dress his Simon Teddy Bear in them. He also loves to play the music on Simon's mobile that played over and over in Simon's hospital room. Samuel loves to play with his Simon bear. He dresses him in a t-shirt that says "extreme" and add sunglasses so his bear looks cool.

All our suffering will be gone one day. As our family focuses on heaven and reuniting with Simon and all of our babies, we know there is hope. As scripture tells us in Luke 6:21, "Blessed are you who weep now, for you will laugh. We will be comforted and fulfilled. In Luke 6:23, Jesus says, "Rejoice in that day and leap for joy, because great is your reward in heaven."

One day I'll visit Koala 2264. I hope that one of his loving nurses will escort me. Some days I'm much stronger than others. I haven't gone yet, but I will. Each day God gives me hope and strength. Each day also has its challenges as well. I recently met two moms who lost their daughters with Trisomy 18 and were in the same NICU. These Body of Christ connections give me courage.

Samuel and Sean build LEGOs for Simon. The finished product is placed proudly on Simon's shelf. Recently, one of Samuel's buddies said, "No offense, but I think Simon really loves LEGOS. Look at all of these!"

Simon's big brothers do love him passionately and miss him terribly. Samuel mentioned how difficult it will be when the school year starts. No longer could he and Sean look forward to their Simon hospital visits. Samuel wished Simon were still in the Koala pod, so he could continue to see him here on Earth. For the boys, it didn't matter that Simon was hospital-bound. He was present physically to them. I mentioned to

Samuel that if Simon still lived in the hospital, Mommy would also still be staying there. He said that would be okay because he'd say hello to me each day on his visit to Simon's room.

Every once in a while I read though Simon's Death Summary. It's heart wrenching, clubbing me with the reality of his loss. Simon isn't here anymore. Yes, he'll always live in our hearts, but we'd give anything to have him here today. His life will always be cherished because he taught us what faith, hope and love really means.

Name: Crosier, Simon
Admit Date: 9/7/10 (it should read 9/6/10)
Birth Date: 9/7/10
Discharge Date: 12/3/2010
Comment: Infant had progressively lower O2 sats (oxygen levels), then progressive decrease in HR (heart rate), held in mom's arms. Pronounced dead by physician at 10:45. No autopsy. Medical Examiner notified and baby released. Case 10-7614.
Birth Weight: 1890 <3%tile (grms)
Birth Gestation: 37wk 6d
Disposition: Died
Birth Head Circ: 32.11-25%tile (cm) Birth Length: 43 <3%tile (cm)
DOL: 88   5
Description: Do Not Resuscitate (We never signed a DNR)

Ann Barnes, RN, co-authored the book Care of the Infant and Child with Trisomy 18 or Trisomy 13, which can be obtained through SOFT at www.trisomy.org. Her daughter, Megan, was born with Trisomy 18 and lived for nearly 20 years. An acute illness and the misuse of a DNR (Do Not Resuscitate) order contributed to Megan's death in 2004. Of the potential misuse of DNRs, Barnes writes in her recent paper *Trends in Health Care for Trisomy 18 and 13*, published in the Spring *SOFT Newsletter*.

"A DNR order can be misused either through error or purpose, which is a breach of trust between physician and parent and can result in death."

In the same paper she writes eloquently about the reluctance of some obstetricians to perform C-sections in the face of a Trisomy 18 diagnosis. Doctors who perform C-sections on Trisomy 18 babies instead of simply letting them die due to the rigors of natural childbirth are true heroes to my family.

"A common trend in obstetrics is to not consider caesarean delivery an option for these babies," Barnes adds. "Thus begins parental realization that health care management might be an issue of concern. More than half of these pregnancies end with elective termination, miscarriage or stillbirth and in both disorders only 5-8 percent of live births (estimated at 1/6000 for Trisomy 18 and 1/10,000-20,000 for Trisomy 13) will survive to celebrate their first birthday. [Carey, JC (2010)] Current information about survivors and care allow parents to make informed decisions, but still today, some parents are not provided accurate information."

A parent should never have to read their child's death certificate. The pain is so deep that I can't possibly describe it. I thought it was horrible reading my Dad's death certificate when he died at age 57. There's no comparison to losing your own child at his age of 88 1/2 days.

I later acquired my obstetrician's notes about Simon. They were clinical sounding words that spread light on the modern medical community's attitude about high-risk pregnancies. These notes were dated June 14, 2010:

"Intrauterine pregnancy with an estimated date of delivery of September 22, 2010, based on early ultrasound. Her estimated gestational age was 25 weeks and five days. If the baby does have Trisomy 18, the prognosis is very poor. Most babies die before birth, or soon after birth, and generally have profound physical and mental defects. While long-term survival is possible, these children are of significant mental retardation, et cetera. The patient was offered the opportunity for amniocentesis, which she once again declined. I had a discussion concerning fetal monitoring and newborn care. Our management would certainly be altered by the knowledge of whether the baby did in fact have a chromosomal abnormality or not, particularly if it was Trisomy 18. Without that

information we would assume the baby has normal chromosomes, and would base any treatment decisions or intervention on the likelihood that the baby has normal chromosomes but would do testing immediately after birth. If there were abnormal chromosomes, it might mean she would need to make a decision about withdrawing care, et cetera."

During my research of other cases involving trisomy children, I came across the tragic story of Barbara Farlow and her daughter Annie. Annie was born, full term, with Trisomy 13. Her parents enjoyed an achievement we could only dream about. They experienced the joy of bringing their daughter home to their Canadian residence. After 80 days of life, growing respiratory distress forced her parents to rush her back to the local hospital. Annie died within 24 hours of arrival. Barb Farlow picks up the disturbing rest of the story in an article she wrote for the *Canadian Pediatric Journal:*

"Annie's death was most difficult for us. She did not have the comfort we would have wished for her in her final days and hours. Annie's siblings rushed to the hospital only to discover that their sister had died just minutes earlier."

Barbara continues Annie's story in another article printed in the American Pediatrics Journal.

"Doctors didn't tell us the truth about what was happening or about the sedatives that they gave her (Annie) against our wishes. We made critical decisions based on misinformation. Much later we tried to get her records so that we could know, finally, what really went on in her last hours. Alas, most of the final records are missing, so we'll never know the cause of Annie's death or whatever treatment existed that might have been to her benefit. The hospital apologized, explaining that sometimes communication for complex children is not as clear as they would wish.

"The gradual realization about how we were deceived and disenfranchised during Annie's last days of life was completely devastating to my family. Five years later. We continue to struggle with anger and hurt. We desperately needed a doctor to look past Annie's genetic label and predicted disabilities and acknowledge and understand

that she was an individual, a very special girl whose family loved her and wanted her to live."

From thousands of miles away, I felt this brave woman's pain. As a parent of a child with life-threatening chromosomal abnormalities, you can easily be led down a path you may not want to go. And trusted medical professionals can lead you in that heartbreaking direction. You have to follow your hearts and be encouraged by Simon's story. Our time was short with him, but it was a joy every day to embrace him. Simon was so captivating and tenderhearted. He felt a strong attachment to us that was so cherished, and always will be.

I braced myself as Mother's Day approached. This has always been a difficult day for me. It's the same day that I've grieved for six daughters lost through miscarriages. Last year, my wonderful husband gave me a beautiful sterling silver bangle bracelet with all of our treasures in heaven — our six girls' names on one side and Samuel and Sean's names on the other side. Still hoping that Simon would be with us as the next Mother's Days approached, Scott had Simon's name lovingly engraved beside his big brothers. The owner at a local jewelry store remembered Scott and our story. He lovingly engraved Simon's name. He was just another Godly person the Lord placed in our path.

Just when you're feeling profoundly alone, God sends you a special person. This time, she happened to be named Betsy. Because of an accident, Betsy is a quadriplegic, confined to a wheelchair. This brave woman told me honestly that she'd prefer to go through life confined to a wheelchair than to be in our shoes. I met this courageous woman at a parent meeting at my son's school. Her words that day inspired me. She emailed me this Mother's Day with a moving poem:

Not till the loom is silent,
And the shuttles cease to fly,
Shall God reveal the pattern

And explain the reason why
The dark threads were as needful
In the weaver's skillful hand
As the threads of gold and silver
For the pattern which He planned.

Author Unknown-

One evening while Samuel attended a birthday party, Scott and I took Sean out for dinner. We needed some special time alone. Babies appeared to be coming out of the woodwork. Our innocent kindergartner made a profound observation when he stated, "When Simon was in the hospital, I never really noticed other babies when I went places. But since Simon went to heaven, I see babies everywhere I go." Then Sean said something that made us re-evaluate our attitude about shrinking away from other babies in public because of the constant hurt.

While we ate our dinner, Sean said: "I think the devil tempts you to look at babies because he knows it will hurt us and it is so painful." Scott and I began to agree with him. Of course, Satan wants to cause us more pain and suffering. But then Simon's beautiful peaceful presence embraced our hearts in his pure love. Without any words between us, Simon's message to us was received and internalized. I smiled at my husband through my pain and patiently explained to our son that our all-loving Lord doesn't want us to give in to that way of thinking. I asked Sean to remember Simon every time he looked at one of God's little children. Simon would want it that way. Our little six-year-old somehow seemed at peace with this answer.

I still have emotional exhaustion at times. It is through Christ that I gain strength. He calls me to do the job He gave me here on Earth. My family also gains strength from the people who continue to acknowledge Simon. The other day, Auntie Judy introduced me to a friend and said, "She has a son, Simon." It was not had a son, she said HAS a son, Simon.

How awesome to recognize him and me as Simon's mother. There are days that I feel good to just cry, and when my tears are not flowing, it's because I'm holding them back when I'm in public. It hurts so much to hold them in. Sometimes I want desperately to enjoy a good long cry. Having two young children to care for, I battle to hold myself together. But sometimes, I'm given the gift of that precious private moment to grieve and talk to my little angel in heaven. After that, I'm fortified with God's grace to be the best mom I can for my two here on earth. Thank God He allows me to make it through each day! Thank God for prayer, a means to cling to Jesus. I believe with all my heart there is no other way to get through this life. I know we all must endure trials and suffering but we can never lose hope in Christ. Through him alone is the light and the way and the only path to be reunited with all of our loved ones.

How could our Simon have had an extra chromosome, I ask the Lord at times. Simon was part of my family. As a mother, I had precious plans for my Simon. My biggest hope was just to love him. We waited so long for our little guy. Samuel and Sean were such awesome big brothers. They were so proud of him. They wanted always to hold him and be involved in his care. There was nothing they wouldn't do for him. This is what unconditional love is, a full-circle experience. Simon was a part of them, and they were a part of Simon. We all wanted Simon, special needs and all! We wanted him just the way he was. As the boys always said, "Who cares about the cleft lip, it makes him cute."

Simon's smile was nothing short of captivating. His big brothers said his smile was even bigger than normal because of his cleft. His big eyes were so beautiful, and they punctuated his calm and peaceful demeanor. His favorite spot was in his family's arms. His love radiated throughout the entire room! Some medical professionals will tell you trisomy babies have no personality because they have no intellect. That's the way people think who have textbook knowledge but no compassion. Any feeling person who had the privilege of meeting or holding little Simon gave testimony to his fighting spirit, loving ways and engaging charm. His primary nurses fought good- naturedly for the special opportunity to provide his daily care. They all loved him!

Listen to the words of his nurse Olivia and decide for yourself if Simon lacked a personality:

"It's indescribable how I felt when I first made eye contact with him," she said. *"We had a unique bond. I always knew what he needed. He would become upset when his O2 saturation levels dropped — but I knew how to calm him and he always responded to me very well. His eye contact was amazing — I always had the sense that he was smiling through his eyes. He seemed like someone much older and wiser than a mere infant. Yes, he was a joyous old soul."*

To mark Simon's nine-month birthday in early June 2011, we went to Simon's grave to release star balloons in tribute to his inspiring example. As Samuel and Sean watched the balloons disappear in the sky, they told us that Simon was grabbing them from heaven. Sean lost his very first tooth that day. To my oldest son, this wonderful milestone was only sweeter because it fell on Simon's special day.

Sean also has built Simon's big, big LEGO house in heaven. It has four floors and lots of room for Simon to play. Sean's Grandpa, and my Dad, "Papa," must be so proud of him because Papa was an engineer. I couldn't help thinking of a favorite Bible verse from John's gospel: "There are many rooms in my Father's house. I am going now to prepare a place for you, and after I have gone and prepared you a place, I shall return to take you with me; so that where I am you may be too."

Simon inspired more miraculous building projects. Our neighbor Karen Smith and her daughter Abby built a brightly colored bridge and named it "Simon's Bridge!" I call it another *Godincidence* because Scott and I had been talking about a Simon Bridge for the previous couple of months. Although our neighbor never suspected our plans, she proudly called us over to look at her project when she completed it. We immediately felt the warmth of God's presence embracing us. Simon's love lives on through those with the love and compassion to continue his work.

CHAPTER 13

What's Simon doing in heaven?

I had another Simon dream. I could see Simon. He was in the Koala room with Daddy kangarooing him. They were both so comfortable in the green recliner. I kept wanting to get closer but couldn't.

The next night, I listened smiling to myself as Samuel asked Sean what Simon was doing in heaven. The boys liked to discuss their brother's big, big house. Tonight they said Simon was blowing a trumpet because he is an angel. Sean added that in heaven there is a classroom, so Simon can learn. Well, heaven is sure to have a golf course, driving range and a windmill, Samuel offered. Then my devoted little Samuel added, "I wish I could be in Simon's house and play golf with him."

With the boys asleep, I reflected on my meeting with my counselor Gail earlier in the evening. Gail was always such a tremendous guide and comfort to my troubled soul. That day she said to me:

"My message is to stay with the truth as you know it, meaning that which comes from within embracing the love of children and of family, and that which comes from without, meaning the information given from caregivers. Be aware of projecting fear, which does not reflect reality. The anxiety one feels from past experience has to be acknowledged but not allowed to become a force depriving us from living life as it is gifted to us from one moment to the next.

"I also advocate self-care. If exposure to situations associated with pain become more difficult than can be managed, pay attention to those messages and make decisions in favor of self-care. Healing takes time. We need to honor the process."

After leaving her office, I felt an irresistible desire to turn into the parking lot of the hospital where Simon had lived his short but eventful life. My heart was pounding, my hands shaking and I felt as if my throat would close down — but I **HAD** to do this. I thought: If I don't do this now, I'll never find the courage to do it again.

I arrived outside his building and looked up to the second floor. There was his room, 2264 Koala. The window to the left revealed the nurses' desk. I didn't care if anyone questioned what I was doing there. Simon's room faced a circular drive that was used for service vehicles and not an entrance to the hospital. It was a small, enclosed area with a medical building on the other side. I gazed up longingly at the window, but I couldn't convince my legs to move.

My imagination, though, was free to leave my body. I could see myself holding Simon in that green recliner chair. He was so snuggled up and comfortable. That room was his room. I wanted to be there so badly again. It was home to us for three months, how could it not be now? I wanted to go inside, but how would I know if one of Simon's nurses was working? Was there a baby in Koala 2264? If so, how could there be? Simon's nurses would say that they had a very hard time seeing another baby in that room. It was Simon's room! They still tell me that they envision Simon and me in there. Even now, when I dial Grandma Lois' phone number, I catch my breath for a moment. The last four numbers are 2264.

During that period, I had another Simon dream. I could see Simon. He was in the Koala room with Daddy kangarooing him. They were both so comfortable in the green recliner. I kept wanting to get closer but couldn't. It was so comforting and awesome to see Simon and Daddy bonding. I would dream this dream over and over again any day if I could! But then the next night, I had a bad dream. I dreamt that I was in a support group for NICU parents who were fortunate enough to bring their babies home. I didn't know why I was there; my Simon's home was in heaven. No one here was crying, but I couldn't stop my tears. They couldn't understand my grief, and I couldn't share in their joy.

We still struggle with the grief, and it is very difficult and heartbreaking. It has helped in our healing process to participate in organizations such as the Fetal and Infant Mortality Review Program (FIMR). After responding to their request for more information about Simon, I was interviewed by a nurse from this organization. This program involves a home visit with a representative who came to interview me about my own personal experience. It was the first time I was heard by someone in a position to make a difference in the community. It was a rewarding opportunity to talk about my pregnancy and personal experiences with the loss of Simon and our other precious babies we lost through miscarriage. We also talked about the services we received and the ones that we wished we would have received. We talked about support and the lack of support from medical professionals, family and friends. I cried the whole interview, and I know that our Lord caught all my tears in a jar.

Scott and I also completed a research project specifically in regards to decision making upon diagnosis of Trisomy 18 and 13. The researcher, Pam Healey, is a developmental psychologist who collected data nine years ago on the experiences of parents at the time of diagnosis of their child. This researcher is now collecting information from parents who have had a diagnosis of Trisomy 18 or Trisomy 13 for their child in the past five years to compare with earlier findings. We chose to participate in this study, partly because the researcher's son, Conor, had been born with Trisomy 18 and died in early infancy. She has walked this journey personally and we were also doing it for Simon. The process seemed therapeutic as we kept our little Simon's legacy alive.

We were asked if we perceived any difference in medical treatment of our child versus the treatment of "a healthy normal baby." We were asked to reflect upon the amount or lack of support we received from medical professionals. This allowed us to finally have a voice. We felt from the beginning that Simon was treated like a hopeless case. It was as if we always had to justify our choices and beliefs. But when it came down to it, we always knew there was only one choice: to be proactive for our son. We were repeatedly told, "Not for Simon." They meant they were more interested in providing "comfort care." This meant that there would be no medical intervention to save life or prolong life.

We have also participated in research for TRIS, Tracking Rare Incidence Syndromes (TRIS) project through Southern Illinois University Carbondale. Simon was on their home page in the summer of 2011. He is also in their photo gallery. TRIS is a project to help raise awareness and provide support for individuals involved in the care of children and adults with rare trisomy conditions. This organization does not include Trisomy 21, which is Down syndrome. There are many groups that do support Trisomy 21.

Finding others in SOFT or TRIS has been helpful. Our family looked forward eagerly to attending our first SOFT conference. Meeting other trisomy families seemed like the best therapy to soften our pain.

In late June, I decided I had to visit Simon's hospital room. I wanted to breathe the air that Simon breathed. This is where he had life on earth, and 2264 Koala was his home. I composed myself and resolutely walked through the parking garage and those familiar doors. As I neared the elevators, I stared at the pictures I saw every day when Simon was alive — a butterfly and a squirrel. I just couldn't bear to take the elevator up to the second floor. I told myself one day I would visit his room inside. But that day, this was far enough.

I returned to my car and looked up to the window of Simon's room. The light was on, and I could see the heat lamp that we would use when we gave him a bath, such a bittersweet memory. Maybe coming here had not been a good idea. I was hurting so badly and missing Simon so much. I had empty arms now and they ached so much for our little guy. As I turned on the ignition, my radio came on and ironically, the song said, "Let my life song sing to you, living sacrifice to reach a world in need. Hallelujah!" Simon has a life song that he will always sing to me!

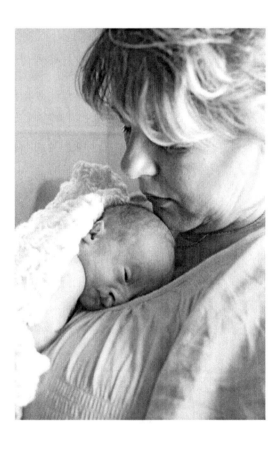

Other losses in my life began surfacing, some from the past and many unhealed experiences. I had to go at my own pace and not allow others to demand that I rush through. Even though the world goes on, people will be selfish and try to hurry you through your grief because it is easier for them. It's not fair, and it actually stunts the growth and healing process. I had to invest my energy in growing and finding peace. I looked forward to my quiet time. While I was vulnerable, it was important to protect my emotional and physical health and be kind to myself.

It's always important to stay away from circumstances or people who hinder this process and make you more vulnerable. It's essential to surround yourself with supportive people who will help you get through this period of rawness. Courage is based on the French word meaning "from the heart." It took great heart to care, to be vulnerable, to love. Praise, honor and celebrate your heart. You have been through losing, surviving, healing and growing.

Our friend Stacy completed a 40-page scrapbook of Simon memories. Stacy once owned a scrapbook store — so you can imagine how awesome it turned out. Such a valued keepsake! It has beautiful pictures of Simon, our family and his nurses. Stacy did a wonderful job inserting our Caring Bridge journals, creating a timeline for Simon's short life. She even included Simon's hair, umbilical cord, his hats, socks and some amazing notes Simon's nurses wrote to him after he passed.

CHAPTER 14

No coincidences with SOFT

"Every life matters. Our kids are not disposable and deserve every consideration. The lesson of our SOFT families that evolves over time is this: the souls and spiritual essence of our children are not disabled. Their physical handicaps exist, but their desire to thrive is not diminished." — Steve Cantrell

So off to the SOFT conference I went, Simon's scrapbook at my side. Stacy worked hard to have it completed before I left for Chicago. I wasn't sure what I would feel or experience, but I was doing it for Simon! His story had to be told. I knew he wanted me to meet other families who lost their trisomy children and those blessed with inspiring survivors here on Earth.

People like Steve Cantrell, who lost his son Ryan to Trisomy 18. I had connected with Steve by email shortly after Simon's death, but this was my first chance to hear his comforting words face to face. "Our son was born Oct. 4, 1985, and lived 8 1/2 months before passing on Father's Day 1986," Steve told me. "We had no idea Ryan had any issues until he was born. At that time, this condition was little known and children did not survive the birthing process. We were all flying by the seat of our pants, including our health care providers."

Steve told me that he and his wife, Peggy, also had to struggle to get Ryan the medical care he deserved. "We became advocates for our son," Steve added. 'We had to convince our medical team we could reach higher. Our kids don't leave us where they found us. During this time, a social worker, Gail Gordon (yes, the same Gail who later became my friend and counselor), who knew our son Ryan, gave us a brochure about a new parent support group in Salt Lake City. We called Dr. John Carey's (the nation's leading physician advocate for trisomy children) number at Primary Children's Hospital in Salt Lake while in the lobby of the St. Louis Children's NICU in St. Louis. To our surprise, he answered his phone and we received factual information, which allowed us to move forward with our medical team."

Harsh words had wounded Steve and Peggy, as they had hurt Scott and me. "Words like grim, bleak, lethal, failure to thrive, or why do you want to do that, he's going to die anyway," Steve elaborated. "Dr. Carey helped us understand what to expect, but also told us there is hope. We also called the parent-founder of SOFT, Kris Holladay, who, like Dr. Carey, amazingly answered her phone for that fateful call. We prayed on the line, shared a long-distance embrace and fed on our new energy to move forward. We were not alone."

Sensing my own nervousness at attending my first SOFT conference, Steve shared his similar initial experience. "My own first SOFT conference was July 1987, after our son had passed," he recalled. "We walked in and my first thought was: 'These people appear to be normal!' This journey begins with self- doubt and only gets more difficult from there. That's why the mission of SOFT is so important — to offer a sanctuary of understanding without judgment and to re-animate our souls. SOFT is tightly woven into the fabric of our lives — we've been involved at every level. Our vow is to pass forward the love and support we received and light a path through the jungle of misinformation.

Steve and Peggy agree there are no coincidences. God connects us at the right time. I will never forget Steve's impassioned defense of the dignity of all life.

"Every life matters," he said. "Our kids are not disposable and deserve every consideration. The lesson of our SOFT families that evolves over time is this: the souls and spiritual essence of our children are not disabled. Their physical handicaps exist, but their desire to thrive is not diminished."

I agree, Steve! How can anyone who meets these precious babies say they are incompatible with life? But Simon had another purpose in his short wonderful life. I would have never had the opportunity to meet wonderful people like Gail Gordon, Debbie Bruns, and Steve and Peggy Cantrell if it weren't for Simon. I'll never understand why we have to suffer so much when we lose someone as special as Simon, but I do know that God's love is constant no matter what happens in our lives. God created us to be in relationship and fellowship with others. God is showing His love for me through the people I meet. Debbie, Steve and Peggy are now walking our journey with us. Lord, please bless us with more trisomy friends.

As I pulled up to the hotel in Chicago for my first SOFT conference, I must admit I was scared. Even though I knew I would see my friends, Debbie, Steve and Peggy, I wasn't sure how it would be to see rare trisomy living children. Would it be upsetting since our Simon was in heaven? Oh, how awesome it would be to bring our little man to a SOFT conference.

The first trisomy child I noticed was outside the hotel in a wheelchair. It was a girl, maybe 10 years old. I was feeling anxious and not sure how I would do this alone. But I wasn't alone. I had Simon in my heart always and was feeling something I had not really felt before. I believe I was feeling Simon's spirit. The rest of our family, Scott, Samuel and Sean, would be traveling to Chicago on Friday with Grandpa Duane and Grandma Lois. Simon and I were on our own until then. Of course, I asked the Holy Spirit to guide us and protect us. Well, I took a deep breath, prayed and got out of my vehicle. I was having many conversations with Simon asking him to guide us and give me Simon signs if this is where he wanted me to be. I proceeded to check in and unloaded my entire family's luggage in the hotel room. With four suitcases and a few other bags, I looked like I was staying for months. I did not know then that I really wouldn't want to leave.

At the luncheon I saw Steve and Peggy right away. I also sat next to Gloria, who lost her daughter Erin to Trisomy 18. "Wow," I thought. "I may fit in here!" I also met many other wonderful parents who lost their children. I will never forget Kris Holladay saying, "Are you Simon's Mom?" How refreshing and comforting to be called "Simon's Mom!" Kris puts together an annual DVD of all of the trisomy children, and included images of Simon in the 2011 DVD. Kris does this DVD in memory of her daughter Kari who had Trisomy18. There was also Barb, the president of SOFT, and her daughter Stacy T-18, who just turned 30 years old in May. What an inspiration Stacy is! Stacy is such a warm, beautiful person. I put my hand on hers and she held on. It felt so good. I think Simon was helping me make all of these connections. I also had the privilege to hold Trisomy 18 survivor Morghan. This beautiful young lady was 14 at that time. Lovely, with captivating eyes, trisomy children may appear smaller than their age, but their beauty is not diminished. It's not unusual to hold a 14-year-old trisomy survivor on your lap.

I realized as I met these remarkable human beings that God has given me a great love for all trisomy children and adults. I felt so honored to hold them and meet them. They're rare, but the experience of meeting these children of God was awe-inspiring and unforgettable!

That first evening at dinner with Steve and Peggy, I brought my Simon scrapbook. I wanted to share my baby with everyone, and these wonderful people embraced the chance to get to know Simon. After all, Simon was with me on this journey. I remember thinking, "This is still your journey because you are part of our family and our SOFT family." At dinner there were two other couples in addition to Steve and Peggy: Frank and Ann Barnes, who lost their daughter Megan T-18, and Sara and Ron Hayes. I sat right next to their daughter Megan Elizabeth Hayes T-18. Megan is now 31 years old. Megan was one of the few born with a normal, healthy heart. Well, Simon and I fell instantly in love with Megan. She was reaching out and holding my hand and constantly smiling at me. Her mom reminded her that she needed to eat her dinner. Megan didn't care about dinner; she was interacting and getting to know Simon's mommy. During my visit with Megan, the Cantrells and Barnes were getting to know Simon and shedding tears on his scrapbook.

Everyone I met was so interested in Simon. This conference was to honor and celebrate all of our trisomy children. It was that evening that I realized I love this new family called SOFT. This family does not change the subject if I bring up Simon. In fact, most of the time, they bring up Simon. The parents wanted to get to know him, and the trisomy children who are still living or who are angels already know Simon. What an amazing connection!

At the SOFT conference is a memory room, a place where families can display pictures and keepsakes of their children who have gone on to heaven. I sat and reflected there alone with Simon.

When I talked with Scott and the boys that evening, I was so excited. I couldn't wait for them to come on Friday. It was a magical place. No wonder these families made these conferences their vacation every year. Each July the conference is in a different city. I learned the 2012 SOFT conference would take place in St. Louis! Okay Simon, are you involved in this decision, too?

On Wednesday at the conference, the SOFT medical director Dr. John Carey looked over Simon's summary medical records. It was so reassuring to have Dr. Carey go through each page and express his thoughts. This dedicated physician started SOFT with Kris Holladay 25 years ago. He is a determined and compassionate medical advocate for trisomy children and their families. He told me he wouldn't have advocated surgery when Simon was only 3 pounds, 12 ounces and was struggling with Trisomy 18-related medical issues as an infant. Dr. Carey agreed with us that waiting until Simon got bigger was a better option. Dr. Carey elaborated that Simon's progress was in line with the growth and weight charts for trisomy children. Those were standards we had never learned about while Simon was alive. Dr. Carey's only question was, "As Simon's pulmonary hypertension was worsening, would that have been the time to intervene with surgery?"

I learned at the conference that many more Trisomy 18 girls survive than boys. There were many sweet girls but, unfortunately, only a couple of full T-18 boys at the conference. For reasons that researchers and clinicians as yet can't fully explain, boys with trisomy abnormalities are more vulnerable at every stage. Females with the full Trisomy 18 typically live much longer.

At the luncheon, I met even more wonderful people, including two moms with living trisomy children. Marta and Susan are part of a trisomy advocacy group called TAG. As advocates for trisomy children and their families, these courageous women and their children know love doesn't count chromosomes. They fight for the world's precious trisomy children. Each of these children has divine value and inalienable human dignity. Just ask God! We became instantly connected. They both listened as I described our positive and negative experiences with medical professionals. They got it! They understood! That evening at dinner it was so reassuring to observe beautiful trisomy kids enjoying the music, dancing and having a great time.

A local Chicago meteorologist presented awards to SOFT children and Rick Santorum, former Pennsylvania senator and 2012 presidential candidate, was also a guest speaker. Senator Santorum has a daughter Bella T-18, who is now three years old. What a wonderful opportunity to meet Rick, who happened to sit at our table. Steve Cantrell, who is also an optometrist, gave Rick sunglasses for Bella. Some trisomy children have light sensitivity so Steve donates sunglasses at each conference.

On Friday afternoon, Scott, Samuel, Sean, Grandpa Duane and Grandma Lois arrived. It was wonderful introducing them to so many new friends in our new SOFT family. Grandma took the boys swimming and then went out to dinner with Grandpa and the boys. It was so thoughtful for them to come. Scott and I had the chance to talk with other parents, and Scott was comforted by this connection of trisomy families. He felt their compassion instantly as I had. We are honored to be a part of SOFT.

On Saturday, we attended the picnic and the Ryan Cantrell Memorial Balloon release. The Cantrells started this ceremony in memory of their son Ryan who had Trisomy 18. Steve Cantrell later recalled the touching origins of this SOFT tradition: "As part of the first SOFT conference, we all stood and shared our stories," he said. "We shared how we had chosen balloons to celebrate Ryan's life with joy. Our pastor had used Jesus' words about Lazarus to 'unbind him and let him go.' The balloons chattered together in the breeze and

were released, rising into a bright blue sky. We were all
transfixed upward, as if to heaven."

As we got on the bus, Alleah, a Trisomy 14 survivor, who
shares the same birthday with Simon, approached us saying,
"Butterfly on our bus." Alleah had no idea how much our
family treasures butterflies. These are our Simon signs! We
released a balloon in memory of Simon and friends Hannah
T-13, Sara T-13 and Molly T-18. Many names were called off
as attendees each released a balloon for a special trisomy
angel. When Simon's name was called, Samuel noticed a
butterfly flying around his head and Simon's blue balloon.

On the bus back from the picnic, Samuel noticed a butterfly
outside his window and shouted this was the same butterfly
that he met at the balloon release. Sean also spotted a
butterfly outside of his window. When we arrived at the
hotel, we noticed more butterflies. As Sean walked off the
bus, butterflies were all around him relaying their special
message of hope to him before disappearing in back of the
bus. Words were not even needed. We all instantly knew that
Simon had greeted us with his lovely sense of humor and
appreciation of beauty.

As we released the balloons and watched them rise toward
heaven, we knew our little Simon was with us. Though his
presence here was short and his loss profound, we've gained
strength and bonded as a family. A bright yellow butterfly
fluttered playfully around us as the daytime colors
disappeared from the sky. Looking at the little inspirational
trisomy faces around us, I was comforted to know Simon
lives on. Our family is blanketed with hope for our future.
Our precious Simon, we'll hold you again in heaven.

We'll continue to recognize and celebrate Simon's life in as
many ways as we can. Grandpa Duane and Grandma Lois
hosted an unforgettable event in memory of Simon. They live

on a golf course in Seneca, Kansas. They planted a beautiful blooming crabapple tree and a marker that is placed next to it with Simon's picture. This picture is very special because Grandma Lois bought this outfit for Simon while he was here with us. It's his favorite color blue, and a car on it says, "Off to Grandma's." Again, as with making the quilt she gave Simon before he was born, this was truly an act of love and an act of faith!

Co-chairs, Duane and Lois Crosier worked very hard to make this tournament happen. We decided to name it the Simon Dominic Croiser 1st Memorial Golf Tournament. All proceeds went to SOFT and TRIS. These organizations increase awareness of trisomy and fund outreach and research.

The night before the big tournament, I met with Dr. Sue Hall. Dr. Hall is the medical director of a NICU and a neonatologist and incredible author of her book, "*For the Love of Babies*." She has such a caring heart and is so compassionate and full of hope. At dinner, which lasted almost four hours, Dr. Hall got to know Simon and even more about SOFT. She is a strong advocate for trisomy children. We discussed her stories of children she cared for. Many questions were answered in my own mind. Life isn't fair, but it's our hope and attitude that pulls us through this journey. Dr. Hall is an absolute gem. We would have been so blessed to have Dr. Hall on Simon's team. We ask God to bless all the neonatologists that care for our smallest human beings. It stormed that night before Simon's event and I continued to pray for good weather. As I closed my eyes that night I was grateful for my new friend, Dr. Hall, I had such peace and comfort overall. Thank you Simon — I wouldn't have met Dr. Hall if it weren't for you little guy.

In her book, Dr. Hall describes the evolution of medical thought on Trisomy 18:

"When I started my training many years earlier, Trisomy 18 was universally accepted to be a 'lethal anomaly,' meaning all babies born with it were expected to die, about half within the first six months, and the other half by one year of age . . . Because their prognosis for what the medical community considered to be a 'meaningful life' was nil, congenital anomalies such as heart defects were not repaired."

Later in her chapter on Trisomy 18, Dr. Hall added, *"Although the life expectancy of babies with Trisomy 18 is almost always severely shortened, this is no longer seen as a justification for withholding medical treatment. Most doctors now agree that babies with trisomies should be offered the same treatment options for their birth defects as babies without a trisomy."*

As we moved into the month of September, we thought often of our little Simon celebrating his one-year birthday surrounded by family and friends with singing, presents and cake. The difference is this year he'll celebrate in heaven.

Samuel and Sean had the opportunity to attend a three-day-long bereavement camp through BJC Health care. It is called Stepping Stones and is run by a very professional staff and volunteers who aim to make the weekend a very memorable and positive time. They understand that children grieve too, and they can be isolated or share their journey with others who have lost a loved one. There are so many activities such as swimming, a carnival and other outdoor games. Samuel enjoyed the carnival the most. He said, "There were games, activities and food, all for free!" They have a memory wall where each child can hang pictures of his or her loved ones and draw something next to the picture. They made stepping-stones, prayer flags, wish sticks and sailboats as mementos. Samuel was speaking to Simon as he placed his sailboat in the water. He said, "Simon, I hope you are watching this." Sean said, "It was so nice to talk about my brother to others who wanted to get to know Simon; people cared about me and my family."

So next time someone tells me that children are resilient and will get over "it," I'll ask them, "Why has Stepping Stones been helping kids for more than 15 years?" They understand children's grief and don't sweep it under the rug. They put the child on a path to peace, understand them and allow them to go through the recovery process.

We believe that by involving our children in the grief process, it can be comforting as a family as well. We've decided to have a birthday party here on earth for our "Master of Ceremonies," Simon Dominic Crosier. Simon's life had such an impact on so many people and those of us here wish to recognize him, always. When special days like this occur, it's time to stop and cherish the moment.

CHAPTER 15

Trisomy 18 facts and impressions

Most babies with the Trisomy 18 prenatal diagnosis are terminated. Among those who are born, some parents choose not to feed them because they are told their baby will die anyway.

With the wonderful, insightful words of Dr. Hall fresh in your mind, allow me to offer a more detailed explanation of Trisomy 18. I'm no doctor, like my compassionate friend Dr. Hall, but my experiences with Simon and the research I've conducted since his passing have filled my world with knowledge about this tragic syndrome. Trisomy 18 children are visitors from heaven and given to us to love and protect here on earth. They may not be able to live in a healthy body, but they're perfect and so pure. These children from heaven love unconditionally and are true angels sent from God. We cherish life, no matter how long. We are grateful for all of our children and promise the Lord we will always protect them from the moment of their existence in the womb. Each human being has value, and only God knows how long these special babies are here on earth before they return to the Most High. There is evidence in certain cases to counter the prognosis of "not compatible with life."

Some facts of Trisomy 18 that I retrieved from the SOFT website (Support Organization for Trisomy 18, 13 and related disorders) include:

Trisomy 18 syndrome (Edwards syndrome) is a disorder of human chromosomes that occurs in approximately one in 6000 live, born infants. Trisomy 18 is due to the extra #18 chromosome. More than 90 percent of infants with Trisomy 18 syndrome will have full trisomy. Seen in Trisomy 18 babies are: congenital heart defects in 90 percent, joint contractures in 10 percent, hearing loss in greater than 50 percent, cleft lip in 5-10 percent. Some common disorders in Trisomy 18 are feeding difficulties, gastroesophageal reflux and apnea. Routine follow up of infants with Trisomy 18 includes child care/anticipatory guidance, cardiac evaluation, hearing test, ongoing support and routine immunization.

Other resources state statistics such as: Edwards syndrome occurs one in every 6,000-8,000 live births in the United States. The child has three of the number 18 chromosomes instead of two. 95 percent with this syndrome die before birth. Between five percent and 10 percent of children with Trisomy 18 live beyond 12 months. About 80 percent of children born with Edwards syndrome are female; it is thought that being male increases the risk of dying from the disorder before birth.

Almost all resources will state that Trisomy 18 is "incompatible with life." These harsh terms scream to me, "completely hopeless." About 90 percent of these patients die before or during birth and 90 percent of those who survive die within the first year. Most babies with the Trisomy 18 prenatal diagnosis are terminated. Among those who are born, some parents choose not to feed them because they are told their baby will die anyway.

In a recent article in the Spring 2012 issue of *The Soft Times*, a vital resource for the trisomy community, Dr. John Carey, MD, SOFT medical advisor, responded to a medical journal article in the American Academy of Pediatrics *Neoreviews*. The article advocates primarily "palliative and hospice care" in treating trisomy babies. Dr. Carey challenged the authors' use of "lethal" as a description indicating that these unique individuals have "no chance for long-term survival." He further challenges the article's closed perspective on quality of life.

He writes: *"The authors accurately mention that 5 percent to 10 percent of children with Trisomy 18 survive the first year of life. It is important to note that in all the population studies that have derived these figures, rarely was* **intensive technological support** *provided for the surviving children with Trisomy 18 and 13. Thus, these 1:10 to 1:20 children celebrated their first birthday with their families because they are likely at one end of the curve of survival. 'Lethal' then in this context is an inappropriate and misleading description."*

He continues: *"At no time is the quality of life of a child with the syndromes and the views of the parents of this quality elaborated on. The reason why this is not discussed is likely because knowledge of the life issues of older children with Trisomy 18 and 13 is inadequately documented in the medical literature."*

I applaud Dr. Carey's findings and disagree passionately with the assessment "incompatible with life." These trisomy babies are visitors from heaven. Every moment with your child is a gift. We wanted Simon, "special needs and all." We encourage parents not to terminate. It is God who determines the number of our days. I also know that the medical community often pushes families toward abortion in these cases. Our compassion must extend to these parents as well. I'm happy that SOFT has welcomed them into our organization.

Psalm 139:15-16 says,

"My frame was not hidden from you when I was made in the secret place. When I was woven together in the depths of the earth, your eyes saw my unformed body. All the days ordained for me were written in your book before one of them came to be. Is the span of life Sovereignty determined?"

Romans 8:28 adds, "*We know that in all things God works for the good of those who love him, who have been called according to his purpose.*"

We don't know when the Lord will call us home. I wanted to write this book and offer my experience to readers who are struggling with a sick child or disheartening diagnosis precisely because I don't know when the Lord will call me home. I pray that we will continue to grow in faith and love for one another. Simon had a profound impact on a large majority of people who followed his journey on earth. I pray that the Lord will change the hearts in order to advance the treatment and care of those with Trisomy 18.

Trisomy 18 support available for parents in the St. Louis area includes:

For parents:

TRIS Project — The TRIS project seeks to increase awareness and knowledge for families and professionals touched by rare trisomy conditions and aims to facilitate improved decision making for optimal services and supports for affected children and their families. I wish I would have known of TRIS during Simon's time with us. The organization displays such hope and understanding of this tragic chromosomal condition.

The TRIS project also seeks to compile a database including information about specialized hospitals, genetic counselors, and other programs and individuals with contacts with families with members with a rare trisomy condition. In turn, these individuals can assist with recruitment of additional families to participate in the TRIS project. www.coehs.siu.edu/tris

TRIS project aims to increase and improve available information concerning the medical, health, educational and support needs of children and their families. An additional outcome is sharing TRIS information with interested professionals including educators, medical specialists and therapists.

Please visit the TRIS site at www.coehs.siu.edu/tris. Check out our precious Simon and the rest of those beautiful trisomy children and adults at www.trackingrareincidencesyndrome.org.

AMEND www.amendgroup.com

Bereaved Parents of America: 314-807-5798

Heartprints, Maggie Loyet: 314-251-6878

Gail Gordon counseling: 314-999-1989

Weavings (Retreat for mothers who have lost a child) www.bjchospice.org 314-273-0776

For children in the St. Louis area:

WINGS, especially expressive therapy: 314-273-0782

Stepping stones www.bjchospice.org: 314-273-0776

Kid's Clubhouse: 314-721-1144

Footprints: 314-268-4110

Annie's Hope, the bereavement center for kids www.annieshope.org

Trisomy organizations for families:

SOFT (support organization for trisomy) www.trisomy.org

TRIS (tracking of rare incidence syndromes)
www.coehs.siu/tris

Noah's Never Ending Rainbow
www.noahsneverendingrainbow.org

A website that describes the heart defects are at
www.pted.org

TAG — Trisomy Advocacy Group,
www.trisomyadvocacygroup.com

Imaging Miracles (www.imagingmiraclestoday.com)
Our Mission: IMAGING MIRACLES GIVES BACK.
We are the ONLY 3D/4D ultrasound service who provides
FREE ultrasounds to educate women who are contemplating
ABORTION. We also provide FREE 3D/4D ultrasounds
for women whose children are given a fatal diagnosis
(Trisomy 13 and 18). Tammy Cowan: 417-861-0071
tammy@imagingmiraclestoday.com

Websites for support:

Hope for Trisomy 13 and 18:
http://www.hopefortrisomy13and18.org/

T18 Moms: http://www.t18moms.com/families.shtml

Trisomy 18 Hope: http://www.trisomy18hope.org/

CHAPTER 16

Coming to terms with grief

*I caught myself looking down to the left imagining I could see him in his crib. I **did** see Simon! I felt him and smelled him. I wanted to pick him up and give him more lovin! I know Simon could see all of us together in his room yearning, silently groaning for his physical presence. Come back, Simon!*

One can become so vulnerable with the passing of a child. We don't pick our relatives. It's not so much about forgiveness — it's about reality. Some people aren't capable of loving, grieving or just having an ounce of compassion. If someone owes you money, and they don't have it, they cannot return it. No matter how right or fair or reasonable it is, they just don't have it to give. Scripture will also tell us that we are to loan without ever getting anything back. We just do things sometimes out of love.

We loved Simon unconditionally, and he offered beautiful, unconditional love in return. He didn't have to do this. An infant capable of loving and expressing himself so clearly was a miracle. He continues to touch so many hearts, and we pray that through him others will feel a connection to their Creator. As we have heard from those who knew Simon best, he was wise beyond his years. If only I could be like him!

As human beings we're not capable of wrapping our hearts and minds around some things. If we could ever understand the "why" of why things happen, our lives might be less painful, but that is not always how the Lord answers our questions. It may not be long before Christ returns. His time is not our time. At that point I don't think I'll have any more questions. This will be the time when everything is crystal clear. But until then, I trust in the Lord.

We'll continue to grieve for Simon for a lifetime here on Earth. The distractions continue to sting, mainly family and friends who remain self-absorbed and walk on by. They never acknowledged Simon's birth or passing.

I'm still learning that it's important to surround myself with people who are supportive and healthy. My counselor Gail asked me the question, "Who is your family of choice?" We can't let toxic feelings grow; we need to keep them where they belong. Our family suffered an emotional injury, and our bodies and souls are healing. It's necessary to trust the process and let it happen. We feel so much pain, sadness, emptiness and helplessness. Once again God gave us our feelings. We need those around us to not stop us from expressing them or feeling them. Right now, we need comfort for our pain. We need to lean on others until we can stand alone.

I lean on people like Tom, who started out as a cemetery gravedigger and over 30 years has been promoted to grounds supervisor of several cemeteries in St. Louis area. Tom shared his personal testimony of divine intervention at our meeting on a chilly November day at 6:30 a.m. at Resurrection Cemetery.

I was there with my son Samuel digging in the dump area looking for pictures of Simon on three bricks that we had displayed at Simon's gravesite. I missed the grounds removal the night before and so I showed up at the cemetery praying that the workers didn't throw Simon's beautiful display away. Samuel got up early and went with me before school. When we got to Simon's grave, we both gasped. The bricks were gone, and I started to sob. It wouldn't have mattered if we lost a few flowers, but Simon's beautiful face was not going to end up in a dumpster if we could stop it.

I continued digging through flowers on the ground hoping to find Simon's display. Nothing!

A well-dressed man pulled up in a truck and asked if he could help. I replied in sheer panic, "I can't find Simon's belongings."

Tom didn't know me, or Simon, but he didn't hesitate to climb out of his truck and up a tall ladder to peer inside a 40-yard wide dumpster. It was completely full, and as Tom looked over the contents, I explained Simon's story. Tom later told me he could see in my face the excruciating pain of losing my three-month-old son. He told me about a recent article in the St. Louis Review that his monsignor encouraged him to read. Although he hadn't gotten to it yet, Tom knew that the article was about a family struggling with the death of a child from chromosomal abnormalities. "You might want to read it," he said. The article he cited was about our family. It was headlined: *Family Shows Love Cannot Be Counted By Chromosomes*. You should have seen Tom's face when I told him it was "our" article.

Energized by this discovery, Tom volunteered to jump in the dumpster and look for Simon's pictures. Tom was late for a meeting at another cemetery, which explained his formal dress. Tom didn't care about his clothes. He later told me the look of pain on my face — and a little nudge from the Lord —told him exactly what he needed to do. Before he could dive into the dumpster, I stopped him with tears of thanks running down my cheeks. What a kind, loving and compassionate man!

Although he was unable to find the bricks, Tom shared with me something even more precious as we chatted at the cemetery as the sun rose over the horizon. He explained that he used to think things happened by coincidence — but not anymore. "God works with us down here on earth," Tom offered. "If you're not an angel —you're a vessel. God uses his people on earth. We may not think we're equipped for the task — but God does. He says to us, 'Just be still and know that I'm God.'"

Tom sees things even more clearly, and so do I. God put us in each other's path for a reason. Tom encouraged us to get a white-bud tree in memory of all our babies in heaven. Tom had a soft spot in his heart for those unborn babies and for our precious little man, Simon. The tree and marker is right in front of Simon's and my Dad's grave. Scott and I decided to have a marker made from Samuel and Sean for their siblings. It reads, "Simon, Sophia and all of our loved ones in heaven. Love, Samuel and Sean."

Tom had tears in his eyes as he told me that his wife had lost two babies to miscarriage. It was many years ago, he said and people didn't talk about it. "It's still painful," he added with a weary shrug. It was another connecting of the dots — a *Godincidence*.

Tom puts it this way: "Nothing is a coincidence to me anymore. There is a connection to God and others orchestrated through our Lord, Jesus Christ. My father used to say, 'If not you, who?'" He said that from his perch high up on the ladder about to dive into the huge dumpster and look for Simon's belongings.

Life pulls us back to living, and we had to leave and go on living once we left Simon's room the day he went to heaven. I lean on people like my friend Ruxandra from my Weavings grief support group. We went to a retreat together that was such a positive experience. Weavings is offered by BJC Hospice to help parents deal with the loss of a child. This lovely woman, who also lost a son, reminded me:

"Is there an answer to the omnipresent phrase, 'It happened for a reason?' As I was driving toward the retreat, I wondered why I had to attend. Soon, I realized I knew the answer. The first evening of the retreat, I studied the weaving on the table in the middle of the room. My son's name caught my eye immediately; however, I noticed another name:

Simon. It seems like a reflection of my son's name, Cosmin, and suddenly I felt a connection between the names. The second day of the retreat, the weavings were rearranged, but our sons were together again! As our sons are together beyond this world, I had to meet my dear friend Sheryl. This was the reason to attend the meeting!

"Since the retreat, our friendship grew stronger and more amazing things happened: the same pair of hands engraved on their stones, the same love for water, and the same desire to see Sheryl and me together. I am wondering what a newborn would have in common with a teenager that lived his life to the fullest. Perhaps Simon needed a big brother to hear stories about life from. One day we will have all of our questions answered. But for right now, our angels are watching over us."

Our family had to leave and go live and walk out of his room for the last time ever! Visiting his hospital room home again and seeing his name on the plaque outside the family lounge were searing memories. Honoring him is what we'll continue to do.

I'll always keep Simon close to me through the meaning of his short life — not his death. Actions such as writing this book and contributing to SOFT lift my heart. Those living children and angels are Simon's trisomy brothers and sisters. Yes, the majority of his biological sisters are in heaven while his two big brothers, Samuel and Sean, keep his legacy alive here on earth.

Life is about being born and dying. When we're faced with a human being and premature death, we long to place meaning on this event. I'm hungry for someone who saw Simon, held him and cared for him. I'm still processing his death and it will take a lot of time. Scott's process may be different than mine — but we still end up in the same place, without Simon.

Having to surrender your beloved son — the one I prayed for with every breath — was heart wrenching. Like Kenny Chesney's song, "I wear the pain like a heavy coat and feel you everywhere I go. The only thing that gives me hope is that I will see you again someday." I have a sorrowful heart now. I'm human. But I do know that our Lord keeps his promises when we just trust him.

I can tell you the peace that I feel when I'm around trisomy families is unexplainable. This is, of course, Christ's peace but also a Simon sign.

The days leading up to December 3, 2011, were extremely difficult. It was so hard to believe our Simon went to heaven almost a year ago. The first anniversary of Simon's death was full of sorrow, but also lifted up to the Lord by the compassion and support from people who knew him here on Earth.

I was so moved by the love Simon's special nurses had for him and still do to this day. 2264 Koala will always be Simon's room to his family and caregivers. Some of Simon's special nurses say that they feel his presence there today and find it difficult to go into his room when they care for another baby.

About a month after Simon passed, I started writing this book. I felt an urgency to express my raw emotions and my journey. When our dear friend Krista inspired and encouraged me to write a book about Simon, a new horizon dawned for me.

Simon brought so much love and joy and touched so many hearts that his story demanded to be told. Trisomy awareness and education and the day-to-day challenges, milestones and hope inspired by his short life required a witness.

Most trisomy families may not get the support they deserve because their child is disregarded or dismissed as a "defect." Or, as in our situation, you enjoy support from some but lack support and emotional engagement of any kind even from some members of your own immediate family. The hurtful words, "at least you had him for three months," leave us numb, not grateful. These "salt-shakers" may not technically know the term "incompatible with life," but they've bought into it! I hope, in these pages, Simon has touched your hearts. I pray you will speak up for these beautiful trisomy children and all the other innocent babies who cannot protect themselves. Never be pressured by medical professionals to terminate these children of God.

The first year without Simon was extremely emotional. Yes, much of the time I was miserable. Even though our family misses Simon dreadfully, because of Samuel and Sean we continue with our holiday traditions and seek happiness among each other. Those traditions now include Simon in everything. Christmas is a time when Simon always will be with Jesus — but he is in our hearts as well. Simon is the bright shining star on top of our Christmas tree with butterfly ornaments. His name and pictures sparkle throughout the tree. He knows the true reason for the season.

I remind myself that Simon is not just part of our family — he is part of trisomy families around the world. Our son has his brothers, Samuel and Sean, but also six biological sisters in heaven to play with him. Of course, babies get "instant heaven," and we know Simon enjoys heaven with his trisomy brothers and sisters as well. Back here on Earth, I thank God I also enjoy the opportunity to meet — through our SOFT family — other trisomy kids and families who are a blessing and inspiration. Being involved with such an honorable, life-affirming organization drives my life forward fueled by positive energy. Special needs children have taken up residence in my heart.

A few weeks ago, Nurse Wendy and I went to see Simon's plaque outside the lounge. His name was on the top of the Koala plaque. We walked past Simon's room listening to a baby crying loudly inside.

The anniversary weekend of Simon's passing came. I prefer to call it an *angelversary*. As a family, we went to visit the

NICU. Nurse Mary was working that evening. She graciously escorted us to see Simon's plaque where we took a few pictures. Dr. Pang saw us in the hall and stopped to say hello. We explained we came to see Simon's name on the Koala plaque, and he mentioned to another physician that Simon had Trisomy 18. Scott chimed in that Simon was a resident in this NICU for 88 1/2 days. "Doesn't sound like 'incompatible with life' to me," he said. Maybe Dr. Pang wondered why we returned to the NICU. Or maybe he realized just how much love we'll always have for Simon. I wish that Simon had been there in person to answer Dr. Pang's questions. If only, instead of an empty room, we were visiting Simon. That would have been a dream come true.

We walked to the family lounge with Mary, where the boys immediately resumed their familiar pattern of asking to play board games and drink hot chocolate. Mary excused herself to check if Simon's room was occupied.

Sean asked for hot chocolate, and I simply said "no," instead of explaining that we didn't have a baby as a NICU patient anymore. The games, computers, TV and hot chocolate were not for us. Samuel made himself at home, sitting down to sign the guest book. Now I'm sure the book is meant for parents and visitors of babies currently in the NICU, but as Scott told Samuel not to sign the book, I thought, "What could it hurt, Simon lived here, too!" I told Samuel to go ahead and just write Simon's name. So biggest brother Samuel wrote Simon's name in fancy letters in the middle of the page. Oh, that beautiful name! Sean, of course, wanted to write Simon's name, too, so he did so across the page from Samuel's.

Minutes later, Mary walked in smiling. "It's vacant — let's go see Simon's room." As we walked down the hall, as we did so many times before, it seemed time had reversed. It was just yesterday that Simon was present and living here in this hospital. Was this day supposed to be our way of achieving closure — or just more grief work?

I can't believe that the same day we're here as a family — the day before Simon passed away one year earlier — his hospital room is not occupied. This is a Simon sign! This is his doing! Our little angel wanted us to reunite and reconnect again in his room. This was his home where we created memories together, where we lived life one moment at a time. It's also the battlefield where we engaged medical professionals about Trisomy 18 — Edwards syndrome — and the care that should have been our son's birthright.

We fought so hard for everyone to see Simon for Simon — as a beloved and respected member of our family. Special needs and all, we wanted him! The times we would hear, "Not for Simon" echoed in my head as we walked down the hall together. Scott, who had always been intently aware of the hall monitors reflecting each baby's vital stats, now stared blankly ahead as he walked toward Simon's room. The boys wanted so badly to run ahead as they once did hoping not to miss a Simon second. But they struggled to be big boys and practiced patience and self-control.

We arrived at the sliding glass doors of Simon's room. Once again it felt as though a knife was taken out of my back and thrust back into my heart — "no Simon in the room." I'm not sure, but it felt like we stepped into that room together — the four of us connected, but separated to grieve for Simon each in our own way. The bittersweet reality of our little man being gone, and the excitement of being in his room again, was hard to put into words. All I know is that each of us, including Mary, felt Simon's real presence. We kept saying this while we stood silently in his room! We felt him. We felt his spirit. We felt Simon.

Right away the boys plopped down on the green couch where I slept many times. They were back home — their other home, because this was Simon's home. They seemed to be waiting their turn to have Simon placed in their loving arms. Sean was absorbing everything in the room, and Samuel wordlessly communicated he was in a very familiar place that he did not want to leave. Since they had not been in Simon's room on his last day, it was so important for them to be here. We always wanted them to remember the good times with their baby brother. This is what they did — had fun with Simon, but Simon doesn't live here anymore.

Samuel and Sean commented that they could feel him as if they were holding him. They smelled him again, and it was a wonderful smell. As we all soaked up his presence, Scott stood close to the sliding glass doors by the same sink where I washed my hands, splashed water on my face and brushed my teeth each day. Scott seemed hesitant, awkward and afraid — as if he was reluctant to open up again and feel. This room is where we lived and breathed Simon's "life." Scott's eyes were full of tears, but he stood so still, as if reality was hitting him fast and hard. "I realize now what Simon was looking at all those times in the room when he seemed to be focused on another world," Scott said with the excitement of someone who had solved a perplexing puzzle. "He was looking at the crucifix on the wall. I never noticed it before."

Mary held my hand as we stood next to the place where Simon's crib had become the center of our existence for three months. I can't explain completely how I felt. But I still feel the electric current of emotions running from my head to my toes. Mary and I often talked to Simon before bedtime. We would just giggle because his clear eyes showed he knew what we were thinking. "Not time for bed yet! I am part of this party, too!" His big eyes followed each and every move. They requested his favorite music and foretold his knowledge and wisdom, saying, "I know what comes next." I caught myself looking down to the left imagining I could see him in his crib. I *did* see Simon! I felt him and smelled him. I wanted to pick him up and give him more *lovin*! I know Simon could see all of us together in his room yearning, silently groaning for his physical presence. Come back, Simon!

Mary walked us out of the NICU to the elevator. We all gave her huge hugs in appreciation of this opportunity. We'll remember this visit for a lifetime. As we silently left the hospital, we got in the car and began discussing the almost supernatural feelings we had just experienced. We are the witnesses to Simon's real presence on this Earth. The next day was December 3. Could we harness the emotions of this special day and put up a Christmas tree in Simon's honor?

In the morning, we went to Kirkwood Farmer's Market and picked out our Christmas tree. We knew Simon was watching us, even as he walked with Jesus in preparation for celebrating the Lord's birthday with him in heaven. The song that kept echoing in my head was Selah's, "I will carry you." As we pulled out our Simon decorations and put up the butterfly ornaments, we again felt him among us. The boys even wanted a little Simon tree, so they put bells and a few ornaments on this as well. Adorning this Simon tree of gold ornaments were the names of the trisomy angels and survivors who we had met.

Simon was always a hat man. We created a Christmas tree of his special hats on the wall. It's a colorful tree because Simon loved his hats in all the colors of the rainbow — just another piece of Simon we'll carry always in our hearts.

In church, they mentioned Simon's name, as is the custom on the one-year anniversary of loved ones. After the service, a woman introduced herself to me. I didn't know her, but she noticed my tears as she sat a few pews behind us. She had no idea this was Simon's *angelversary*. This brave woman shared that she lost two children many years ago. Her son had lived only a week. He would be 50-years-old now. Her daughter only lived a half-hour, and would today be around that same age. Her eyes were brimming with tears and she admitted she still longs for her children. I know this emptiness in my heart

— like the small opening in Simon's tiny heart — will always hurt. For this mother and me, grief will last a lifetime until we are reunited with our children someday.

One of the ornaments containing Simon's picture came with a message I'd like to share. It was a gift from our dear friend Jackie.

Merry Christmas From Heaven...

I still hear songs,
I still see the lights
I still feel your love on cold wintery nights
I still share your hopes and all of your cares

I'll even remind you to please say your prayers
I just want to tell you, you still make me proud
You stand head over shoulders above all the crowd
Keep trying each moment, to stay in His grace
I came here before you to help set your pace
You don't have to be perfect all of the time
He forgives you the slip, if you continue to climb
To my family and friends,
Please be thankful today
I'm still close beside you,
In a special way
I love you all dearly,
Now don't shed a tear
Cause I'm spending my
Christmas with Jesus this year

John Wm. Mooney, Jr.

Wow, how awesome to be spending Christmas with Jesus! As much as we want Simon here, he is in his eternal home and waiting for us. God doesn't want anyone to perish, for He is the enemy of death.

But right now — we're still here on Earth. It may not be our time yet, but we want to be ready. Scripture says we do not know the day or the hour when Christ will return. None of us has a guarantee for tomorrow. I do know that God's will for me is to celebrate His son's physical birth and look forward to his return.

My destiny is to look into my beloved Simon's eyes again. I know that this Earth is not my eventual home. How glorious it will be to finally meet my Maker! What if this is the day I am reunited with Simon and all of my babies? What if Christ returns today? Wow, I can only imagine!

I can feel God embracing me as I embraced Simon. I'm still being taught a lesson of love, faith and hope. Only through the Lord was I able to surrender my son, and God continues to carry me forward. On my own, there are days that I can't put one foot in front of the other. Other times, I can feel Simon as if he is still in my arms, as if he is still in my womb. This is my son staying close to me. This is his mother needing that bond. Simon is coming with me everywhere I go. Even though I had no choice but to let him go physically, he'll always be in my heart. His wise spirit lives on.

Simon's purpose was accomplished. Many hearts were touched and souls were saved. Simon taught me how to die. I'll be forever grateful to my son who prepared my heart and mind.

My broken heart is now a bigger heart. My love for trisomy children and those with special needs is a gift Simon left for me here on Earth. My wise son taught me to look for a deeper purpose.

I am Simon's voice. His name is Simon. He is not a syndrome. Only negative people and Satan himself can try to rob me of my peace. Do I still experience anxiety and deep sadness? Without a doubt! But through prayer and Simon's continued presence through constant signs, I carry my cross each day. My son's love lives on through others and those with the love and compassion to continue his work.

Simon taught me that the quality of life is measured by love. I thank God for Simon's special doctors and nurses. Simon knows who they are. Yes, we grieve, but others will show their divine love by sharing in our journey. God made us to be in relationship with others. Debbie Bruns led Simon's family to a new trisomy family. It's a family so giving and genuine. Thank you, Debbie. I can only imagine what it will be like to meet my heavenly family where trisomy abnormalities no longer exist.

We know that God uses all of life's experiences to strengthen and guide and correct his people. Our finish line is death and the celebration at the end of the race is heaven. As advocates for our trisomy children, we speak for those who can't speak. Jesus keeps me strong, and the angels and signs he places in my path minister to my soul.

I don't know why Simon had Trisomy 18, but I know that God loves Simon. My son still has a purpose! Every time I have the opportunity to tell Simon's story, I pray the Lord will touch another heart with the knowledge that each life matters.

I believe the Lord has strengthened my marriage through this struggle. No, it hasn't been easy; just ask my husband. But we take comfort in knowing that the Lord guards marriage against harm when faith is present. We continue to hang on. Scott has shown grief in ways different from mine. He is upset that people don't acknowledge Simon. But my stoic husband's day isn't ruined when he encounters a baby Simon's age or an expecting mother. He reminds me that he is a guy, and has never been pregnant before. Scott focuses on providing for our family. At times his deep sadness rushes out in tears and feelings of frustration. I pray for Scott to be honest with Jesus and not rush through the pain.

We're not home yet, but while we're here, we must fight for what is right. We'll achieve long-term justice only by speaking up for those who can't speak for themselves. We must respect each and every life, no matter what the syndrome or diagnosis that person faces. The diagnosis is not the person. The time they exist here on Earth does not define their value. These "divine appointments" have immeasurable value to the Lord and an eternal life as glorious as any King, president, movie star or star athlete. Our beloved son was never a syndrome. His name is Simon, and we anxiously await our reunion day in heaven with him and our Savior!

AFTERWORD

By Grandma Lois

After we lost our precious grandson, Simon Dominic Crosier, we really wanted to plan an event in his memory and at the same time to raise money for research of Trisomy and outreach to help other families. Simon's parents and brothers suggested a golf tournament. We both felt this was a great idea since we live on Spring Creek Golf Course here in Seneca, Kansas. Seneca is 90 miles from the Kansas City International Airport. My husband, Grandpa Duane immediately contacted the club pro and there was only one date available in the summer, August 20, 2011. We went with that date and Duane started contacting hole sponsors and sent out fliers and e-mails. I contacted businesses for silent auction items and hole prizes.

The month before Simon's golf tournament we went to Chicago for the SOFT conference. We really gained a greater understanding of Trisomy and enjoyed meeting so many wonderful families, those who still have living Trisomy children and those who have lost their trisomy children. We know how special our grandson is and so are all these children with Trisomy. At that time we knew that we wanted to offer hope for all Trisomy children and their families. We agreed to donate Simon's golf tournament proceeds to SOFT (Support Organization for Trisomy and related disorders) and TRIS (Tracking Rare Incidence Syndromes).

We were so pleased and grateful for all the support of this small community, a town of 2,000 people. We only had one business turn us down. There was 38 hole sponsors at $100 each, 27 four-person teams at $200 a team, 25 items for silent auction, 10 hole prizes donated and an auctioneer donated his time as well. In addition, we had a foursome - "Team Morghan" sponsored by a SOFT mother, Faye Kaufman for her daughter Morghan. Steve and Peggy Cantrell - who lost their son Ryan. Ryan had Trisomy 18 also. They are another SOFT family to donate to the tournament as well. A local Topeka, Kansas Neonatologist and author made donations, too. Dr. Hall is also an advocate for Trisomy children and spent time the weekend of the golf tournament with Sheryl, Simon's mommy.

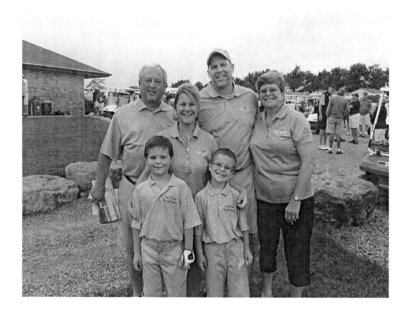

The day of the tournament started out a little cloudy and chance of rain but it turned out to be a beautiful day. We thanked Simon for that, for his "Simon signs" of butterflies were everywhere. Scott, Simon's father introduced the family before the tournament and announced what the proceeds would be used for. Simon's big brothers, Samuel and Sean, golfed so well. It made them feel very good. Everyone who played or helped with the tournament was very upbeat and positive and really made the tournament a great success. We were very pleased with how well it went and were happy we could do something in memory of our precious grandson, Simon Dominic Crosier. The total proceeds with matching from Simon's Daddy's employer totaled $9,000.

We always prayed for the maximum time with Simon. I will always treasure the time I had holding, loving and having sleepovers with my grandson in his NICU room. Simon touched so many lives and taught us what quality of life really is. It is measured by love.

Simon loved life, was always so alert and had a beautiful personality with a bright spirit. He will always be perfect in every way and we continue to celebrate our beloved grandson always until we all meet again in heaven.

We love you Simon and miss you so much.

Hugs and Kisses,

Grandma

AFTERWORD II

by Deborah Bruns, Ph.D. Principal Investigator,
Tracking Rare Incidence Syndromes (TRIS)
project, Southern Illinois University Carbondale

It started with a phone call. Sheryl Crosier contacted me for information about the Tracking Rare Incidence Syndrome (TRIS) project. It was shortly after Simon's passing. Sheryl was full of emotion, telling me about Simon's medical issues, growth and, above all, his personality. She told me about the rollercoaster ride of medical crises and interactions with medical professionals as well as her family's needs. I was drawn in from the beginning. This was a story that needed to be shared. Though it won't bring Simon back, it speaks to his legacy. Eighty-eight and a half days of life is more than a number. It is a testament to his will to share his time with those who became a part of his life in obvious and less obvious ways.

I didn't have the opportunity to meet Simon but I feel I knew him. Sheryl's verbal descriptions and photos opened a new world for me. I had met many families through my involvement with the Support Organization for Trisomy 18, 13 and related disorders (SOFT), but this was raw and real. By this I mean his passing was recent and Sheryl wanted to know if she made the appropriate decisions on Simon's behalf. She also wanted to make a difference or rather have Simon make a difference. Through our phone calls and meetings in winter 2010 and spring 2011, we forged a connection that went beyond Simon to the trisomy community. I encouraged Sheryl to attend the SOFT Conference in July 2011. She came along with her husband, Scott, and sons, Samuel and Sean. I was excited to see the other families welcome her with open arms. Sheryl found her place and was more motivated and determined to bring this book to fruition.

My initial encounter with children with a rare trisomy condition was when I was an Educational Therapist at the New York Founding Hospital in the early 1990's. I had two girls in my classroom, both three-years-old at the time, with full Trisomy 18 (like Simon). There was another four year old in the program with the same diagnosis. When I looked for information on the newly introduced World Wide Web, I was greeted with autopsy photos and the term "incompatible with life." The irony of having three living youngsters with different skills levels and personalities was not lost on me. I read the scant information I found and used my teacher instincts to plan activities and work with them to encourage their development. A few years later I began my doctoral studies and once again fell into the trisomy world through an online listserv (Our Kids). A mom from Australia with a son with Trisomy 18 mosaic was a frequent poster. Her messages fascinated me as she chronicled her son's medical issues, her interactions with medical professionals and her advocacy on his behalf. She soon began several listservs for the rare trisomy community. I joined and learned what no textbook or research article could teach me. I learned compassion, perseverance and the bonds that link parents and families who are on this journey.

The TRIS project began in 2007 with online surveys to collect information medical conditions, developmental milestones, educational and therapy needs, and family support. Nearing the end of 2011, there are approximately 450 families participating in the project from around the world and representing children who lived up to two months and long-term survivors. Diagnoses include all types of Trisomy 18, 13,

9 and 8. Several publications with TRIS project findings have been published (Bruns, 2011a, b; Bruns, 2010; Bruns, 2008; Bruns & Foerster, 2011) and others are in various phases of preparation. What is critical to highlight is the more positive outcomes in these studies as compared to previous literature (e.g., Parker, Budd, Draper, & Young, 2003; Pont, Robbins, Bird, Gibson, Cleves, & Tilford, 2006). Recently, a more favorable perspective has begun to emerge about the care and treatment for newborns and children with these conditions (Glassford, 2003; Kosho, Nakamura, Kawame, Baba, Tamura, & Fukushima, 2006; McGraw & Perlman, 2008; Mercurio, 2011; Shaw, 2008; Walker, Miller, & Dalton, 2008). It is also important to note the initial work of Dr. Carey and his colleagues (e.g., Baty, Blackburn, & Carey, 1994) as paving the way for the TRIS project and improved outcomes for these special children.

I'm Not a Syndrome — My Name is Simon offers a strongly personal perspective on the worth of a life and those he touched. Reading this book and coming away with its messages of hope and resolve offer powerful testimony how one life can impact those closest to him and others on a similar journey. Simon was a gift for 88 ½ days and will continue to be so for parents, family members and professionals living and working with these wonderful children for many, many years to come.

Trisomy friends

Simon, and children like him with Trisomy 18, face many challenges and also bring much joy to their families. Simon left an indelible mark on Sheryl, Scott and his brothers. He showed them unconditional love, acceptance and determination. It is not over-reaching to say that Simon's trisomy brothers and sisters have the same impact on their respective families. The comments below share this sentiment:

"Since Molly passed away, we — and this 'we' includes more than just my husband and me, it extends throughout our families — try to love others unconditionally." (two months, deceased)

"Erin made a profound impact on our entire family. I think we all became better people for having known and loved her." (six months)

"Kayden is a very valuable part of our family. He has taught my husband, myself and our two sons so much about true love, patience and strength when we thought we had none...We are better people and a closer family because Kayden is in our life." (10 years old)

"Morghan heightens our senses to life's experiences. She gives definition and purpose to everything we do and enables us to see and appreciate well beyond what we could before her or would without her. Morghan has made Mark and me better people ... She, in her quiet, nonverbal manner, teaches us, loves us unconditionally." (15 years)

"We loved her dearly and so feared Megan might not survive. She was the little teacher in our family who gently touched our hearts. How blessed our family was to have had her for as long as we did." (19 years old, deceased)

"Megan has filled our lives with so much unconditional love and joy... has helped us be more understanding and compassionate in all aspects of our lives. She has taught us tolerance and extreme patience. Megan has brought many wonderful people into our lives that we may never have had the opportunity to meet." (30 years old)

"Caleb had the sweetest spirit, the purest heart and a contagious smile. He meant the world to our family and friends — even to total strangers. Caleb was full of so much unconditional love. He taught us how to appreciate the simple things in life, like the shadows on the ceiling from the ceiling fan." (2 year old, deceased)

Stacy changed our lives. Thirty years ago we were told our beautiful baby girl had already outlived her life expectancy. We were devastated. We held her, loved her unconditionally and connected with other families in SOFT. They are our support our friends and our extended family. (30 years old)

The worth of a child can't be measured by his diagnosis — just as the worth of an adult cannot be measured by his occupation or value of his house. There is a need to step back from evaluating a life based on what the individual can and cannot do or provide to society. A life should be viewed and valued for its positive impact on others as described here. Simon touched many just as children like him affect those around them in constructive and affirming ways.

It's equally important to raise the awareness of professionals of the value of Simon and other children with Trisomy 18. Much of the literature points to severe delays, multiple medical conditions and limited lifespan. This is true for some but not all children in this group. There needs to be a shift to the living, to the survivors. Concomitantly, medical, educational and other professionals such as respiratory therapists and speech and language pathologists must increase their knowledge of common conditions and their implications for treatment and services. Anecdotal evidence and a small but growing research base is providing information with the potential to increase the likelihood of treatment and improve overall quality of life. New ways to address respiratory and cardiac problems such as those Simon experienced hold promise for enhanced outcomes no matter how long or short in days, weeks or years, for example.

While the prevailing perception has been to limit treatment due to the poor prognosis for children with Trisomy 18, steps are being taken in a more positive direction. Proponents, including parents, medical professionals and other interested parties, are pushing for greater understanding of the medical conditions associated with Trisomy 18, as well as the likelihood for improved outcomes. Many children are celebrating their first birthdays and beyond. This is documented both anecdotally and in the research literature. Yet, without a concomitant increase in timely information related to daily care and medical needs, recommendations for care will continue to be based on the diagnosis, not the individual. This information sharing must extend beyond professionals across medical fields but also to those in training to be neonatologists and pediatric cardiologists and other specialists. Without raising awareness of the range of needs as well as outcomes, forward movement in terms of encouraging treatment will not proceed.

A related issue is working with parents and medical professionals to fully understand the parameters of Do Not Resuscitate (DNR) orders. In some cases, doctors make decisions on behalf of parents and their children with Trisomy 18, resulting in not providing emergency care when parents desire that type of intervention for their infant, child or adult child. Decisions about care and quality of life are not intended to be made based on a diagnosis but on evaluating many factors with the most central resting with the individual's family with the support of the medical team rather than at cross purposes or, sometimes, without parent input. Even with a prenatal diagnosis, parents may not fully comprehend the scope of a DNR order for their child. The larger concern is reducing the likelihood of requesting a DNR order for a child with Trisomy 18 based on diagnosis alone.

Positive news can be found in discoveries by those at the forefront of improving perceptions about children affected by Trisomy 18. Within the past decade, a recommendation for six-month checks for Wilm's tumor has been gaining attention. Wilm's tumor is a type of cancer of the kidneys that largely affects children with genetic conditions or birth defects. Immunization schedules are another area of interest. The majority of infants and toddlers with Trisomy 18 are small in size. This, coupled with respiratory difficulties, puts this group at risk for adverse reactions to immunizations. The timing of shots should coincide with the child's weight rather than chronological age to minimize the likelihood of complications. An additional condition often found in children with Trisomy 18 is light sensitivity. The use of sunglasses alleviates much of the problem, but this can be a challenge with younger children who may be difficult to fit or need adult assistance to keep their sunglasses on. There are also feeding issues common to this group that warrant further study. Children with Trisomy 18 display low muscle tone, which affects swallowing and other aspects of eating and drinking. In order to receive the necessary daily nutrition, oral feedings are often inadequate. The use of feeding tubes assist intake but can cause other problems. Additional digestive system issues may also be evident and require attention.

Taken together, the voices of parents presented here and the need to raise understanding of professionals about children with Trisomy 18 points to a larger need to value and nurture this group no matter the lifespan or presenting medical problems. Each child must be seen as an individual. An individual with Trisomy 18 writes his or her own story that we parents, friends and professionals are fortunate to have a part in and learn from. Sharing cases such as Simon's is critical to increase awareness of medical complications and, more importantly, family needs.

Thank you, Simon, for letting me be part of your story. You have taught me more than I can ever teach others about rare trisomy conditions.

REFERENCES

Baty, B., Blackburn, B., & Carey, J. (1994). Natural history of Trisomy 18 and Trisomy 13, Part I: Growth, physical assessment, medical histories, survival, and recurrence risk. *American Journal of Medical Genetics, 49,* 175-188.

Bruns, D. (in press). Birth history, physical characteristics, and medical conditions in long-term   survivors with full Trisomy 13. *American Journal of Medical Genetics Part A.*

Bruns, D. (2011). Presenting physical characteristics, medical conditions and developmental status of long-term survivors with Trisomy 9 mosaicism. *American Journal of Medical Genetics Part A, 155*(5), 1033-1039.

Bruns, D. A. (2010). Neonatal experiences of newborns with full Trisomy 18. *Advances in   Neonatal Care, 10*(1), 25-31.
Bruns, D. A. (2008). Pregnancy and birth history of newborns with Trisomy 18 or 13: A pilot study. *American Journal of Medical Genetics Part A, 146A*(3), 321-326.

Bruns, D. & Foerster, K. (2011). 'We've been through it all together': Supports for parents with children with rare trisomy conditions. *Journal of Intellectual Disability Research, 55*(4),   361–369.

Glassford, B.A. (2003). Case study in caring: Trisomy 18 syndrome [electronic version]. *American Journal of Nursing, 103*(7):81-83.

Kosho, T., Nakamura, T., Kawame, H., Baba, A., Tamura, M., & Fukushima, Y. (2006).   Neonatal management of Trisomy 18: Clinical details of 24 patients receiving intensive treatment. American *Journal of Medical Genetics A, 140A*:937-944.

McGraw, M. P., & Perlman, J. M. (2008). Attitudes of neonatologists toward delivery room management of confirmed Trisomy 18: Potential factors influencing a changing dynamic. *Pediatrics. 121*, 1106-1110.

Mercurio, M. (2011). The role of a pediatric ethics committee in the newborn intensive care unit. *Journal of Perinatology, 31*, 1-9.

Parker, M., Budd, J., Draper, E., & Young, I. (2003). Trisomy 13 and Trisomy 18 in a defined population: Epidemiological, genetic and prenatal observations. *Prenatal Diagnosis, 23*, 856-860.

Pont, S., Robbins, J., Bird, T. M., Gibson, J., Cleves, M., & Tilford, J. (2006). Congenital malformations among live born newborns with trisomies 18 and 13. *American Journal of Medical Genetics Part A, 140A*, 1749-1756.

Shaw, J. (2008). Trisomy 18: A case study. *Neonatal Network, 27*(1), 33-41.

Walker, L. V., Miller, V. J., & Dalton, V. K. (2008). The health-care experiences of families given the prenatal diagnosis of Trisomy 18. *Journal*

For additional information regarding Trisomy 18 survival rates, common medical conditions and treatment, refer to the articles below:

Bruns, D. A. (2008). Pregnancy and birth history of newborns with Trisomy 18 or 13: A pilot study. *American Journal of Medical Genetics Part A, 146*, 321-326.

Bruns, D. A. (2010). Neonatal experiences of newborns with full Trisomy 18. *Advances in Neonatal Care, 10*, 25–31.

Carey, J. (2010). Trisomy 18 and Trisomy 13 syndromes. In S. B. Cassidy & J. E. Allanson (Eds.), *Management of genetic syndromes*, 3rd edition. Hoboken, NJ: Wiley-Blackwell.

Courtwright, A. M., Laughon, M. M., & Doron, M. W. (2010). Length of life and treatment intensity in infants diagnosed prenatally or postnatally with congenital anomalies considered lethal. *Journal of Perinatology, 31*, 387-391.

Crider, K. S., Olney, R. S., & Cragan, J. D. (2008). Trisomies 13 and 18: Population prevalences, characteristics, and prenatal diagnosis, Metropolitan Atlanta, 1994–2003. *American Journal of Medical Genetics Part A 146A*, 820–826.

Graham, E. M., Bradley, S. M., Shirali, G. S., Hills, C. B. & Atz, A. M. (2004). Effectiveness of cardiac surgery in trisomies 13 and 18 (from the Pediatric Cardiac Care Consortium). *American Journal of Cardiology. 93*, 801-803.

Irving, C., Richmond, S., Wren, C., Longster, C., Embleton, N. D. (2011). Changes in fetal prevalence and outcome for trisomies 13 and 18: A population based study over 23 years. *Journal of Maternal Fetal Neonatal Medicine, 24*, 137–141.

Janvier, A., Okah, F., Farlow, B. & Lantos, J. D. (2011). An infant with Trisomy 18 and a ventricular septal defect. *Pediatrics, 127*, 1-6.

Koogler, T. K., Wilfond, B. S. & Ross, L. F. (2003). Lethal language, lethal decisions. *The Hastings Report Center, 33*(2), 37-41.

Kosho, T., Nakamura, T., Kawame, H., Baba, A., Tamura, M. & Fukushima, Y. (2006). Neonatal management of Trisomy 18: Clinical details of 24 patients receiving intensive treatment. *American Journal of Medical Genetics Part A 140,*:937–944.

Lakovschek, I. C., Streubel, B. & Ulm, B. (2011). Natural outcome of Trisomy 13, Trisomy 18, and triploidy after prenatal diagnosis. *American Journal of Medical Genetics Part A, 155*, 2626-2633

Lin, H., Lin, S., Chen, Y., Hung, H., Kao, H., & Hsu, C. et al. 2007. Clinical characteristics and survival of Trisomy 18 in a medical center in Taipei, 1988-2004. *American Journal of Medical Genetics Part A, 140*, 945-951.

Maeda, J., Yamagishi, H., Furutani, Y., Kamisago, M., Waragai, T., Oana, S. et al. (2011). The impact of cardiac surgery in patients with Trisomy 18 and Trisomy 13 in Japan. *American Journal of Medical Genetics Part A, 155*, 2641-2646.

Vendola, C., Canfield, M., Daiger, S. P., Gambello, M., Hashmi, S. S., King, T., Noblin, S. J., Waller, D. K., & Hecht, J. T. (2010). Survival of Texas infants born with Trisomies 21, 18 and 13. *American Journal of Medical Genetics Part A, 152A*, 360–366.

Walker, L. V., Miller, V, J. & Dalton, V. K. (2008). The health care experiences of families given the prenatal diagnosis of Trisomy 18. *Journal of Perinatology 28*(1), 12-19.

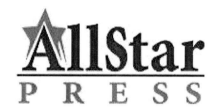

Books That Change Lives

ALL STAR PRESS PUBLICATIONS & WEBSITES:

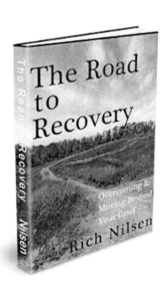

ARE YOU SUFFERING FROM THE LOSS OF A LOVED ONE?

"THE ROAD TO RECOVERY"

by Rich Nilsen

Rated 5 Stars on Amazon.com

Help is here if you are suffering the loss of a loved one. As helpful as friends and family can be, often times they cannot provide the understanding you need because they don't know what you are going through. Rich Nilsen lost his college sweetheart and wife of four and a half years in a commercial airline crash in 1997. She was only 27 years old.

In "The Road to Recovery" Nilsen discusses that you come to a crossroads in your life when you lose someone very dear to you. To help you choose the right path, it is vital to read the work of someone who knows full well the deep sorrow you feel and can provide both comfort and practical advice that works. That is where this book comes in.

Testimonials

"The contents are amazing and profound. Your words rang loud and true when I read them. Wish I had found this book earlier." - Terry Welch, sister to Michael Ryan lost on Comair flight 5196, Aug. 27, 2006.

"I just read The Road to Recovery. It was so informative. I am founder and director of a bereavement support group for parents who have lost a child." - Ann Carruci, HANDS (Healing and Nurturing Distraught Survivors)

"We would love to get a copy of The Road to Recovery and see if we can incorporate it into our resource materials in some way. Again, I want to thank you for developing this material and for your incredible effort to reach out to those suffering from the 9/11 disaster." - April Naturale, New York State Director, Project Liberty.

"Be assured that we will have your support guides distributed to those who have lost a loved one in the tragedy of Sept. 11th. Thank you for all you have done to help alleviate some of the pain borne by loved ones of those who died on September 11th [2001]." - Rev. Msgr. Gregory Mustaciuolo, the Secretary to His Eminence, Edward Cardinal Egan.

"This book contains so many insightful, appropriate and helpful ideas and suggestions. God bless you." - Kelly Markillie, pastoral counselor at The Cathedral of Christ The King, Atlanta, GA.

"I lost my son in the World Trade Center [911] and I found your book so comforting." - Patricia Noah, mother of Leonard M. Castrianno, Cantor Fitzgerald, 105th floor World Trade Center.

"The Road to Recovery" is jam packed with helpful advice and resources to guide through this turbulent time, and make sure you get on the road to a better life. Healing is around the corner.

If you or someone you love is dealing with sorrow, this book will be of great comfort and offer invaluable bereavement advice that you can begin to apply today. Each day can and will get easier. Download this book to your eReader or PC today.

http://www.griefhelp.org

http://twitter.com/griefhelp

EBOOK NOW AVAILABLE IN ALL FORMATS

Available in both English and Spanish

"The Road to Recovery: Overcoming & Moving Beyond Your Grief" is also available in Spanish on Amazon.com

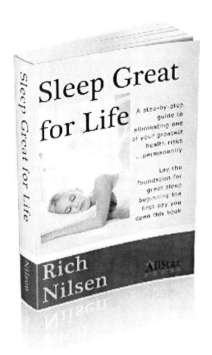

SUFFERING WITH INSOMNIA?

Do you suffer from one or more nights per week with Insomnia? Is getting to sleep oftentimes difficult? Or do you wake up in the middle of the night and then have trouble falling back to sleep? If any of these situations occur more than one night per week, then you are suffering with sleep-related issues. There is help.

The solution is found in "SLEEP GREAT FOR LIFE" by Rich Nilsen, and this powerful e-book is available in all ebook formats.

www.sleepgreatforlife.com

twitter.com/sleepgreat

NOW ONLINE in all ebook formats

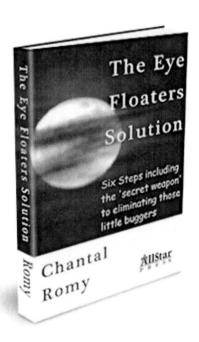

"The Eye Floaters Solution" by Chantal Romy

COMING SOON TO AN ONLINE
BOOKSTORE NEAR YOU:

"Monica Loves the Movies" by Steve Wolfson

"My Wild Ride: The untamed life of a girl with no self-esteem" by Susan Bump

"Angel Gabriel: A True Story" by Joy M. LaPlante

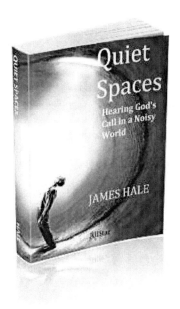

QUIET SPACES: Hearing God's Call in a Noisy World

By James Hale

Learn to hear God's calling in your life and apply it successfully to your day job. This book includes a bonus 45-day devotional.

Here is an excerpt of this wonderful book:

I think God is pretty much the same now as He was thousands of years ago. He hasn't upgraded His technology. For most of us, He tells us of our callings not through shouts, but through whispers—just like He did with Jesus. And if we aren't paying attention, we will miss them.

There are two types of callings: the loud, drama-filled, unmistakable directions that make the good Bible stories, and the quieter, more subtle, personal nudges meant for one person. These latter ones are not intended for public viewing. They are soft, personal, one-to-one messages from God to someone for whom He has a purpose. Maybe for you.

Of the two, the quieter ones are the more common, but less understood. These are ones that Jesus and so many others experienced in biblical times...and today. It's these quieter callings I want to talk about for a moment. These are much more subtle than the dramatic ones. These messages cascade gently down from on high, and we DO hear them, but we often do not LISTEN to them.

The great physicist Albert Einstein understood the goodness of God—like most people do—but he also understood the quietness of so many of God's greatest works and how we often miss his messages or think he's being elusive or tricky. Einstein observed that "God is subtle, but He is not malicious." Yes, God is deep and profound, but not devious. Understanding God often baffles and confuses us, but there is no deception, no false path. God places the cookie jar within our sight, and invites us to stretch to reach it, without any traps in the way. He calls to us in quiet, subtle ways, and none of His callings are evil or misguided. There are no tricks, no deceit, no misdirection.

The softer callings are a lot like snow falling. Think about the first real snowfall of the year. (My apologies to those of you in warmer climates.) This snow coats everything. You can't avoid it. If you're outside, the flakes start landing on you right away. Nothing outside can escape the snowfall: the mighty oak can't, small bushes and shrubs can't, and all of the mundane landscape features like mailboxes and sidewalks get covered, too. My old junker car gets buried, and sometimes the pesky neighborhood dog accumulates a few flakes. And as the snow falls, the world takes on a beauty, a depth, a mystery I may not see at any other time. There will be trees I notice that I have walked past a hundred times before, but have never seen. There will be an infectious charm in what is typically passé, and the naturally alluring features of the world will look dressed for some truly special occasion.

Some callings are the same way. They are gentle. The messages are everywhere. And they turn everything into glory. But we don't always hear them. Sometimes we see the beauty of freshly fallen snow, and sometimes we sigh and just break out the shovels. We often miss the beauty of our callings, too. I wonder how many people Jesus called to discipleship who were too busy to hear the message. I think about those people a lot. I bet there were potential apostles who never knew Jesus was there. Jesus said, "Come follow me," but the message didn't register with them. After all, they were busy. Sometimes God calls us, and He just gets a busy signal, or the ringer is turned off.

Have you ever heard snow fall? It does make a sound. It's about the same level of intensity as most callings. In contrast to the bells-and-whistle callings, the majority of callings are subtle, non-dramatic, and quiet. At least on the outside. But inside they work on you. They drive you to see God's intent. But regardless of the manner in which they are delivered, all callings do one thing: They bring you into a closer relationship with God. It's not about the work you do; it's about how the work works on you. A true calling changes you. If the job is one where you can see God, it is a calling, and it is your earthly purpose. To be able to see God through your work is the greatest gift anyone could have. A king, millionaire, bank president, or lottery winner could not do any better.

Learn how to hear and better apply God's purpose for you in both your life and workplace. Order *"Quiet Spaces: Hearing God's Call in a Noisy World"* today on Amazon.com or at AllStarPress.com

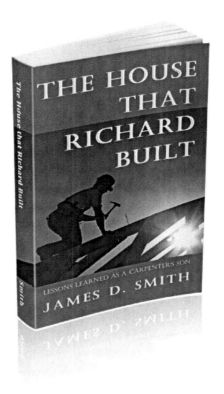

THE HOUSE THAT RICHARD BUILT:

Life Lessons as a Carpenter's Son

By James D. Smith

Rated over 4.5 Stars on Amazon.com

This is a powerful and moving book from Kentucky Pastor James D. Smith that details the life lessons he learned as the son of a carpenter. It is currently available exclusively through Amazon.com for the Kindle eReader, Kindle App, and online through the Kindle Cloud.

It's true that we are all carpenters; we are all building something. We are building families, marriages, careers, relationships, and legacies. Do we have the right type of tools and instruction to build the life we want? You can learn about these power tools for life in the new e-book "The House that Richard Built."

Order it today on Amazon.com or at AllStarPress.com

"I'm a Not a Syndrome - My Name is Simon"

1st Edition published in e-book August 29, 2012

1st Edition published in print October 24, 2012

© Copyright 2012 ALL STAR PRESS